HEAD INJURY AND THE FAMILY:
A LIFE AND LIVING PERSPECTIVE

Arthur E. Dell Orto, Ph.D., C.R.C.
Paul W. Power, Sc.D., C.R.C.

Copyright © 1994
PMD Publishers Group, Inc.
PO Box 4116
Winter Park, Florida 32793

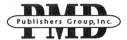

Opinions and views expressed in this book do not necessarily represent those of PMD Publishers Group, Inc. nor does it serve as an endorsement for those views or opinions.

ISBN: 1-878205-61-7

Library of Congress Catalog Number: 93-85847

Printed in the United States of America

TABLE OF CONTENTS

Table of Contents iii

Preface vii

Chapter 1 A Perspective on Head Injury:
           The Titanic Revisited 1

           Personal Statement:
           After Winter Comes the Spring 8

           Set 1: Curing Traumatic Brain Injury 13
           Set 2: How Long? How Old? 13
           Set 3: Is the Person with a Head
                  Injury More Important than
                  the Family? 14
           Set 4: Who Should Pay for the Care
                  of a Person with a Head Injury? 14
           Set 5: My Family and Head Trauma:
                  Where Do We Stand? 15

Chapter 2 Impact of Head Injury on the Person 17

           Personal Statement:
           Homecoming of a Brain Injured Veteran 27

           Set 6: Head Trauma and the Family:
                  How Would You Like to be
                  Traumatically Head Injured
                  Like Me? 32

Chapter 3 Impact of Head Injury on the Family 35

           Personal Statement:
           Almost a Vegetable? 46

           Set 7: Prime Of Life 52

Chapter 4   **Family Considerations in
Adjustment to Head Injury**............................ 55

Personal Statement:
...I'm Just Waiting for the Worst to Happen 66

Set 8: Rain or Shine 68
Set 9: I Am in Love with a Stranger 69

Chapter 5   **Family Assessment** 71

Personal Statement:
...We're Tough 79

Set 10: Good Feelings, Bad Feelings................. 81

Chapter 6   **Head Injury and Family Interventions** 85

Personal Statement:
...One More Burden 97

Set 11: Enough is Enough 99

Chapter 7   **The Crisis of Head Injury in the
Family: A Helping Approach** 103

Personal Statement:
Life is Never Uncomplicated 110

Set 12: Fragile: Handle with Care 116

Chapter 8   **Loss, Grief, and Head Injury** 119

Personal Statement:
For Better or For Worse 129

Set 13: Why Us? 133

Chapter 9   **Group Counseling: A Resource for
Persons and Families Challenged by
a Head Injury** 137

Personal Statement:
Better Than Being Alone 147

Set 14: Common Pain, Mutual Support 148

Chapter 10   **Respite Care: Its Critical Role in
Coping with Head Injury** 153

Personal Statement:
Things Change 164

Set 15: How Can I Help? 168
Set 16: Who Needs this Kind of Help? 168

Chapter 11   **Alcohol and Disability: A Head Injury
Perspective** 171

Personal Statement:
Attitude is Everything 182

Set 17: One for the Road 184

Chapter 12   **Hope, Need, and Reality** 191

Personal Statement:
Making Dreams Come True 198

Set 18: Trauma Helicopter 199
Set 19: Justice and Injustice 200

Appendix A   **Support Groups and State Associations of
the National Head Injury Foundation** 205

Appendix B   **Selected Resources** 209

Appendix C   **Selected Books and Periodicals
Related to Head Injury, Disability,
and the Family** 217

Appendix D   **Selected Films and Videos on
Head Injury** 223

Appendix E   **An Educational Program for Families
of Persons with Head Injury–A
Practical Application of Head Injury
and the Family: A Life and Living
Perspective** 227

Index   233

PREFACE

It is estimated that more than two million individuals per year will experience a head injury from varied causes, such as automobile accidents, blows to the head, falls and physical abuse (NINDS, 1989). With advanced medical technology, an increasing number of persons will survive the trauma, but at what physical, emotional, financial, and familial cost? Since head injury exists within a family context, careful consideration must be given to the short-term, as well as long-term impact upon individual family members, as well as the total family system. When head injury occurs, the person's family, as well as significant others, are dramatically affected. Complex problems are posed for family members who are experiencing the effects of a head injury, while coping with uncertain treatment outcomes, and adjusting to losses associated with a traumatic life event.

Even though the family struggles to maintain its equilibrium while bearing the day-by-day burden of coping with head injury sequelae, it can still be a vital force in the treatment and rehabilitation process. According to Sachs (1991), the family must be included in treatment planning and implementation if rehabilitation is to be effective for all the survivors. Because the family has an important role in the rehabilitation process, greater attention must be given to its current and future needs.

This book focuses both on how the family can adjust and survive the trauma related to head injury, as well as become a partner in the treatment, rehabilitation and adaptation process. This perspective is developed by emphasizing important topics which include:

- the impact of the head injury on the person
- the impact of head trauma on the family
- family considerations in adjustment
- assessment
- interventions
- family crisis
- group counseling

- respite care
- alcohol abuse
- loss and grief
- hope and optimism

The format of this book is a combination of original material, personal statements and structured experiences. The original material is presented as a reflection of our thoughts based on our own professional experience, our prior publications (Power & Dell Orto, 1980; Power, Dell Orto, & Gibbons, 1988), and interpretations of the works of others. The personal statements written by family members, survivors, and significant others, put into perspective the issues relevant to treatment, personal adaptation, and family survival. These statements represent a special contribution by our colleagues and friends, and create a framework for the material in this book. The Structured Experiential Tasks (SETs) are designed to enable the reader to participate in personalized experiences which heighten one's awareness of the impact of head injury on the family. These experiences have been systematically developed by the authors with a focus on the major themes from each chapter. An important resource in this book is the material contained in the appendices which include resources related to head injury and of potential interest to survivors, family members, and professionals.

The theme of this book is directed toward a family-oriented treatment and rehabilitation perspective. We believe that a family perspective is essential in order to create a viable approach that supports families living with the complexities related to a head injury. It is from this perspective that the reader will discover ways to involve the family in treatment and also learn some answers to the following questions:

1. How does the family influence the adjustment of a family member who is living with a head injury?
2. What are the resources and potential resources of the family during the treatment and rehabilitation process?
3. How can health care providers assist the families to maintain balance in their lives as well as attain a reasonable "quality of life."

In this book, the terms "health care professional" and "helper" are used interchangeably to identify those people who, in some way, include in their job or life responsibilities an involvement with the family. Physicians, nurses, social workers, rehabilitation counselors, psychologists, family advocates, physical therapists, occupational therapists, peer counselors, speech pathologists, audiologists, and most importantly, survivors, their families, and significant others are some of the groups for whom this book is intended. All of these people have, in the estimation of the authors, an excellent opportunity to assess family dynamics as they affect the person with a head injury, to provide support for the family, and to share information about effective coping strategies and community resources. The book also originates from a multidimentional perspective which is essential for a meaningful understanding of what is important to the survivors of a head injury and their families.

The actualization of this book is a result of the combined efforts of many persons. We would like to thank Marilyn Price Spivack who gave us the inspiration, Janet Williams for her encouragement in the early stages of the development of the book, Brian McMahon who pointed the way, Valerie and David Collins who are making the Journey, Paul Murphy and Keith Smith, survivors who did the impossible, and Michael Bales and Laura Bales who put it all into perspective. A special acknowledgment is made for Carol Keydel who facilitated the development of several personal statements and Cheryl Gagne who shared a unique perspective. We would also like to acknowledge the support of Ken Paruti who put the administrative structure in place for the project, Susan Cannata whose skill put the manuscript in order, Cheryl Thomas whose help with the appendices is greatly appreciated, Barbara Power whose feedback was most valuable, Stephanie Howell who did the typesetting and layout of this book, Dennis McClellan of PMD Publishers Group who supported our efforts, and finally our families who were most understanding during the process.

Arthur E. Dell Orto
Paul W. Power
Boston, Massachusetts 1993

REFERENCES

National Institute of Neurological Disorders and Stroke (1989). Interagency head injury task force report. *National Institute of Health*, Bethesda, MD.

Power, P. W., Dell Orto, A. E., & Gibbons, M. (1988). *Family interventions throughout chronic illness and disability*. New York: Springer.

Power, P. W., & Dell Orto, A. E. (1980). *Role of the family in the rehabilitation of the physically disabled*. Austin, Texas: Pro-Ed.

Sachs, P. R. (1991). *Treating families of brain-injured survivors*. New York: Springer.

1

A Perspective On Head Injury:
The Titanic Revisited

A Perspective On Head Injury: The Titanic Revisited

No words or feelings are adequate to express the comprehensive sorrow, pain, anger, disappointment, and hope shared by persons and families changed and challenged by the impact of a head injury.

While the reaction of the family varies according to the severity of the head injury, subsequent losses, and potential for rehabilitation, a common denominator for families is that they have been changed, forever. This change is a result of complex and long-term demands placed on the family system. These demands can rapidly deplete the most resourceful families, magnify its difficulties and result in intergenerational, emotional, physical, as well as financial bankruptcy.

The evolving challenge for health and human care is to become more aware of and responsive to the needs of families challenged by a head injury as well as the many other complexities related to the life and living experience.

The reason this is critical is that most health care and rehabilitation systems are not primarily designed to meet the changing and emerging needs of families. This deficit often adds to the stress, strain and distress experienced by the family forced to let go of a loved one and renegotiate a relationship with an individual who is not the person they knew, loved and cared for prior to injury. This stress often occurs during the initial nightmare of emergency room and medical procedures when families or significant others are frequently abandoned, left to fend for themselves, and forced to rely on their meager and faltering resources. The result is that families are terrorized and put at emotional risk in most hospital and health care environments that are far from hospitable. This emotional desolation is often the starting point from which families are launched into a potentially unending nightmare that may cover weeks, months, years, or a lifetime. While the sudden onset of a traumatic brain injury can not be undone, the support needed by families to cope with a head injury certainly can be improved.

Anyone who has born witness to the life or death of a loved one in a trauma center can attest to the aloneness that is often part of these environments. Support, caring, and understanding at this point in time is critical because it marks the beginning of a long journey that may be characterized by a loss, potential gain, and increased vulnerability.

Personally, we do not believe that health care and rehabilitation systems are uncaring by intent. We do believe that due to the enormity of the demand, the complexity of the problems and the opportunity and pressure for profit, these systems may be forced by default into compromised roles.

The erroneous assumption made by most health care and rehabilitation systems is that somehow, and at some time, the family is going to be willing and able to bind its resources and respond to role changes and demanding expectations in order to facilitate the rehabilitation of a family member or "loved one." Unfortunately, not all persons who are head injured are "loved ones." There may be a family member who has been characterized by dysfunction and this person may have had a central role in causing the family distress. It is important to consider this perspective when attempting to access the family as a resource in the treatment and rehabilitation process.

This point was illustrated by the following statements by persons faced with the head injury of a family member.

1. What a living hell! My son is one case where we would have been better off if the doctor let him die on the highway. They actually put his brain back in his head and now I must live with a partial person who is killing me emotionally, just as he did before the accident. We would both be better off dead!
2. This is not my wife! I did not plan on living my life with someone I do not know or care about any more. Before this, I was thinking about a divorce—now, I am planning one!
3. It is your fault. You bought the motorcycle even though we knew he had a drinking problem. I'll never forgive you.

As intense and as real as these statements are, they can be balanced by examples of families who were able to make more optimistic statements, but still may be in need of support, encouragement, and understanding.

1. I will do anything to help my son. Any problem can be solved, any burden can be managed.

2. My wife is very important to me. Even though she is not what she was, she was once a great wife and mother.
3. We decided to do the best we can and rely on our friends, family, and faith.

While these statements are reflective of different frames of reference, they indicate the significance of the history of familial interaction and how values and traditions can determine the willingness of families to engage in the health care rehabilitation process.

For the family of a person living with a head injury, the treatment and rehabilitation process is a sequence of demands, challenges, disappointments and rewards. The major question to ask is where, when and how are families going to get the support, resources, encouragement and skill they need to negotiate the emotional and physical perils of the health care and rehabilitation process? Fortunately, there has been the emergence of new ports in this storm which certainly make the process more reasonable, bearable and survivable. (See Appendix A and B.)

While there is an explosion of research relative to head injury and there are more programs, hospital units, rehabilitation centers as well as more services in general, there is much more to be done on all fronts. However, our frame of reference on where the field is today goes back 15 years when in Boston, one of the great medical and rehabilitation centers of the world, there were inadequate programs to meet the needs of a young women who had sustained a severe head injury. When referrals were made to some several rehabilitation programs, the mother of this young person visited the facilities and stated that they were not adequate, and, in fact, they did not understand the needs of her daughter or a family with a brain injured member.

This mother, driven by her love for her child, told us that she would change the system and do something about it. In fact, she did. In 1980, Marilyn Price Spivack co-founded the National Head Injury Foundation and in the process she created a new dimension to meeting the needs of those persons and families challenged by head injury. The point is that it took a concerned, caring, energetic, dedicated mother to begin to challenge and change the system. However, prior to 1980 there were persons with a head injury and their families cast adrift in a sea of confusing uncertainty and hope based upon desperation. In 1994, many problems related to living with and in spite of a head injury have been solved, many created, and some are yet to emerge. The focus of this book is to better understand the enormity related to coping with head injury within a familial and life and living context while being sensitive to the emerging, changing needs of those persons and families challenged by an experience and process that, if unchecked, can deplete, consume and destroy most family systems.

One of the major challenges of coping with trauma, loss or head injury is that people and families are unprepared for and unaware of the potentially harsh reality that can impact their family. Consequently, most people are vulnerable because they live their lives based upon untested belief systems, and are shocked when their beliefs are not validated by reality. They believe that people who are ill and disabled should be taken care of, persons with head injuries given quality health care and families provided with support and concern. These are beliefs which make people feel good about their humanity and create a frame of reference within which they can interpret the world around them.

However, a critical incident in life and living occurs when individuals and families are "put to the test" and must make the choice to translate beliefs into action.

For example, how many people live their lives:

- believing that their family loves them so much that they will always take care of them regardless of the problems related to a traumatic injury?
- making promises to each other that they will never leave each other no matter what challenges or traumas they have to deal with?
- hoping that because they have been self-sacrificing for their children that they in turn will be equally devoted to them when they are in need?

When these beliefs are challenged by the reality of illness, disability and loss in general, or head injury in particular, individuals and families are often faced with an opportunity to validate their beliefs or recognize that their beliefs may have been untested myths.

Head injury has the potential of challenging familial belief systems because of its complexity, intensity, irrationality, and long-term nature. These characteristics force families to not only examine their belief and value systems, but also to make major structured adjustments to accommodate the emerging needs of the family member who has experienced a head injury.

The success or failure of structural adjustments in the family and its members is often determined by the pre-injury life-style of the family. Unfortunately, most families do not prepare themselves for the possibility of a head injury challenging their resources. Consequently, families are often forced to be reactive to head injury because they have not based their beliefs and values on a realistic frame of reference. For example, some people believe that if you take care of yourself physically, by eating the proper food and exercising, that you will live a long, healthy life. The reality is that this *may* happen, but the harsh reality is that no matter what we do in this life, we and our loved ones will become ill, disabled, age, and die. Few of us think of this reality beyond the cognitive level. We all know this in varying degrees, but most of us are unable to translate it into a functional belief system which permits us to look at life, illness, and head injury from an "opportunistic perspective." For most people, their life is spent building financial security. They think that if they save money and develop wealth, they will be able to insulate themselves from the ravages of illness and disability as well as its concomitant financial burdens.

While it is true that financial resources can make the process of head injury more bearable, money cannot insulate people from the emotional burdens relative to head injury. An additional dimension to the myth of financial security is that in today's economy, many families are forced to spend their resources on long term care and create a situation of intergenerational, emotional, and financial bankruptcy. As one parent stated, "I did not save and sacrifice all of my life so that I could pay for coma management for my child. I want to leave something for my other children and my grandchildren apart from bills and resentment." This statement is poignant because it focuses on the intense emotion of a life being dramatically changed and the rupturing of a dream. The harsh reality is that in today's society, the astronomical costs related to health care of persons with a head injury have not only created a crisis for most families, but an opportunity for the public and private sector to take a leadership position in helping individuals and families living the head injury experience to attain and maintain a reasonable "quality of life.".

In order to better understand and cope with the complexity related to a head injury we must think of it as a condition of living which will give families and society a chance to validate humanity by practicing what we say, demonstrating what we believe, and putting into practice religious principles which help people, gracefully and with dignity, make the transition from health to illness, illness to disability, loss to gain and desperation to hope.

Just as the Titanic was considered to be unsinkable and invulnerable, many families believe that their "family ship" can weather any storm. The problem is that head injury and other life challenges represent those unpredictable "icebergs" that can impact families at any time during the life span, at the most unexpected moment and often have irreversible consequences. The challenge is to help families negotiate the perils of life, living and loss without losing their perspective, purpose, sense of self, and their soul. No burden is too great that it cannot be carried. The challenge is to have a meaningful destination and not to make the journey alone.

The following personal statement, "After Winter Comes the Spring," by Michael Bales, Sr. is a perspective on a long challenging journey driven by love, hope, and personal concern. This personal statement is followed by discussion questions and several Structured Experiential Tasks (SETs) which are designed to explore personally and experientially selected dimensions of the head injury experience within a life and living perspective.

PERSONAL STATEMENT

AFTER WINTER COMES THE SPRING
by Michael W. Bales, Sr.

For the past nine years, I have lived a life few people, if any, would choose to live. A lifestyle forced on me by events beyond my control. I am a guardian and caretaker for a person with a disability who is also my legal spouse, and she is a victim of traumatic brain injury. Stress has been so great at times I have felt like running away and giving up. Yet I have accepted my fate and met it head on and through it all received many rewards and a feeling of satisfaction. I have learned many lessons and matured from my experiences.

One of the most difficult disabilities for family members to adjust to is traumatic head injury. Unlike other disabilities, head injury is caused by an injury to the brain normally during the prime of the victim's life. This injury alters the victim's behavior, personality, and cognitive functioning for life. Life after head injury is never the same, for the victim or their family.

In October 1983, Laura Jane Wilson and I moved in together in my home in Hardin, Missouri. We enjoyed a very loving relationship and planned to marry in the summer of 1984. Our life together was to soon be tragically altered forever.

On June 8, 1984, I received a phone call at my place of employment from the Missouri State Highway Patrol. The patrolman notified me that my fiancee had been in an automobile accident, and I needed to immediately proceed to Research Hospital in Kansas City. I arrived at the hospital in time to see Laura being carted from the Lifeflight helicopter to the Emergency Room and she was not recognizable. I was later informed by the doctors that she had sustained numerous injuries with the worst being a fractured skull and massive brain damage. She was not expected to live.

This began a long emotional journey for me. Laura did not die, but she also did not wake up; she was in a coma. Doctors gave her little hope of ever awakening from the coma. She stayed in a comatose state for three months. During this time, I could not grieve since she wasn't dead, but I also could not feel relief since she was not awake. I kept remembering how on television programs coma victims eventually wake up and say, "Where have I been?" I hung to this delusion and hope for months.

Eventually, in September 1984, Laura did awaken from her coma. She did not awaken as they do on television. She awoke like a newborn baby unable to feed herself, talk, walk, or control her bowels and urine. She did not know anyone or even where she was. This was quite a shock to me, but I hung onto the belief she would still be the Laura I knew before injury.

In November 1984, Laura entered extensive rehabilitation at The Rehabilitation Institute, Kansas City, Missouri. She made slight progress during her five month stay. I worked with her and learned what the therapists were doing to help her progress. In February 1985, discharge planning began for Laura since the professionals all felt she had reached her potential. At the time, she was functioning like a two-year-old child and it was being recommended she be placed in a nursing home.

I would not accept this prognosis and started designing a plan to bring her home and continue rehabilitation. Wanting Laura to have a warm home environment, I decided I would attempt to rehabilitate her at home by hiring home health aides to do therapy with her, and be her companions while I was at work. The plan also incorporated into it outpatient visits at The Rehabilitation Institute for continued professional therapy, and guidance from them to use on what techniques to use. I named this experimental program: The At-Home Rehab Program. The Institute and the Ray County Probate Court both approved my plan in February, thus on March 8, 1985, Laura was discharged to my care and she came home with me.

When Laura came home in March 1985, she was unable to talk, walk only with assistance, and functioned at the level of a two-year-old. She was totally dependent on the aides and myself. I was placed in the roles of being her nurse, teacher, caregiver, and in many ways, her parent.

The first year Laura was home I lost many aides who quit due to Laura's tantrums. For Laura, frustration from not being able to communicate, her physical injuries, and her struggle to accept her injury caused her to have frequent tantrums. This is normal for most survivors of traumatic head injury. She would physically attack her aides and me at times. I finally designed a behavior modification system using rewards and a frustration bag for her to hit that slowed down these attacks and eventually ended them completely.

In October 1985, the Ray County probate Court gave us consent to legally marry so we could establish legal rights to each other. Under Missouri law I needed this marriage to be appointed her guardian. The guardian determines where the disabled person lives, and is responsible for their care and well being. Laura was functioning at a three-year-old level at the time of the marriage, thus it was not a normal marriage. Being Catholic, the marriage was not recognized by our faith nor did we want it to be since it was done for legal reasons. I must admit a part of me still hoped that maybe the marriage would change Laura back to who she used to be, a hope I had not yet given up on, but was starting to.

Laura made remarkable progress in 1986 and 1987. Tantrums ceased, and her level of functioning constantly increased. Professionals were amazed at her progress and started asking me to share my techniques with them. Laura, and the At-Home Rehab Program became the focus of several state-wide and national news articles, and even appeared on the KMBC-TV news as a story by Mr. Bob Werly, health reporter.

During those years, major emotional changes took place in both Laura and I. Finally I had come to accept Laura would never again be the person I loved and knew before her accident. She had started calling me Daddy, which at first I would not accept from her. We sought out psychological assistance and through such it was documented that indeed Laura viewed me as her parent figure. Dr. Marie Bickett, Ph.D., helped guide us through this change in our relationship, to learn to accept it, and live with it. It was painful, but I adjusted my love for Laura to match her love for me, and became comfortable with it.

As a result of the success of my program and my caring for Laura, after the injury I was elected to the Board of Directors of the Missouri Head Injury Association in June 1986. I was appointed chairman of their Legislative Committee in January 1987 and became the key lobbyist in the state for head injury. I have served as the leading spokesperson in the state for survivors of head injury and their families as President of the Missouri Head Injury Association from September 1987 to October 1988.

Today, Laura is functioning at the level of a sixteen-year-old, can talk some, walk, run, and is independent in many ways. Testing has shown her with an IQ of 73, considered a miracle by professionals who thought she'd never reach this level. She continues to progress, though we know she will never again be who she was prior to the accident. The At-Home Program is now used as a model by one service provider company.

We are very comfortable with our relationship as it has grown to be, and very happy in the way we live. I continue to serve the Missouri Head Injury Association as immediate past president, and Laura attends many functions sponsored by them. We've had a pending divorce on file since 1988 and have not finalized it due to a state law that automatically removes me as her guardian upon dissolution. A state law that we and several advocacy groups are working to repeal through the legislature.

Many people have said to me, "I couldn't have handled it, how did you?" Well, I almost didn't. There have been times I have been close to leaving. I've had three relationships with women I fell in love with only to lose them all due to my continuing to care for Laura. In spite of all the changes, and stress of the past six years, one thing has not changed and that is my commitment to provide Laura as normal a life as possible. I made this commitment in 1984 and I cannot break it for any reason. That has been the factor that keeps me doing what I do, for to me a promise is not given to be broken later, it is meant to be kept. I continue to keep my promise, and will, and through it all there are rewards and growth for me as a person. To me, there is a great deal of satisfaction seeing Laura achieve things we were told she never could, and seeing her smile when she does them. Her being happy, and having as normal a life as possible, makes it all worthwhile.

Reflections

It has been nearly nine years since that day in 1984 that altered our lives forever. There have been many changes since that day. There continues to be change; for life is full of changes for us all.

In years past, we used to at this time of year reflect on memories of before the accident. Now it seems like there never was a "life before accident" and we reflect on "life after injury." Over the years here we have learned the NHIF motto of "life after head injury is never the same" is definitely a true statement but also is the new motto, "life after head injury is worth living."

Little did we realize that out of our tragedy would come a new life and challenges no one could imagine. Laura's life ended; Laura's life began. Like the phoenix arises from its own ashes, Laura has been reborn in a new form. She continues this transformation and growth. Far beyond the most optimistic prognosis of professionals in 1984 and 1985; Laura continued to grow and improve. In fact, Laura has now been adjudicated partially incapacitated, thus she has had some of her legal rights restored.

This has had its costs. We've paid the price in many ways. We've had battles to fight and win besides her rehabilitation and growth. We've undergone changes most persons could not cope with and many cannot understand.

Throughout it all we've had the support and understanding of special people who have helped us maintain and go on. The list of special people is very long so I cannot name each of you but you know you are one. Each year we celebrate Laura' rebirth and new life and show appreciation to you by hosting the annual Life Celebration.

I have entered relationships with women to see these relationships fail due to the life we lead. Yet, I have been fortunate to share life the last 18 months with Debra Cantrell, who has lost a loved one to head injury. Her own personal experience with head injury in her family has made her more understanding of our lives here and has helped the relationship work to this time. There are no guarantees this will continue to work, yet, one must recall there are no guarantees in life. We live the best we can each day.

People have come and gone in our lives. The truly special people remain. To you we owe a debt of gratitude. Your contributions to the success of this program and Laura's life is priceless. No one can truly imagine the real value of friendship and love to a survivor of head injury and their families. There is no price one can set. It is one of the greatest gifts one can give.

Life after head injury is not easy for the survivor or family nor will it ever be. We have to adapt to lifestyle changes one cannot imagine until they experience it. We enter a world no training can prepare you for. We live lives that are no longer "normal." We do not relate well to the "normal world" anymore for its does not exist for us any longer. Those who lead so called "normal lives" frequently view us with suspicion and cannot understand our lifestyles. Yet the word "normal" defined means, "conforming to a norm," and a norm defined means "something generally expected." Head injury has no norm. Each survivor is different with some similarities. We are still just learning about head injury, its affects on the survivor and the family, and the most knowledgeable professional will admit these facts. We are the pioneers in this field and our experiences may set the "norm" for future survivors and families yet to enter the world of head injury.

We are fortunate here. We have adapted to the changes and became comfortable with them and live life the way that works best for us. The way it is for us no matter what other people think. We are a nonconventional family but a family none the less. You are a part of this extended family. God has blessed you with that special quality to care about others. We are thus blessed by your presence in our lives.

It has been a long curvy road to this point but you have helped make the journey one worth traveling. Thank you.

DISCUSSION QUESTIONS ON THE PERSONAL STATEMENT "AFTER WINTER COMES THE SPRING"

1. If you were engaged and your fiancee had a traumatic brain injury, what would you do? What would your family suggest?

2. If your daughter or sister was engaged and her fiance had a severe brain injury, what would you advise her to do?

3. If she said she wanted to call off the marriage, what would you say?

4. If your son was engaged to be married and was brain injured, how would you respond if the future in-law wanted to proceed with the wedding?

5. If your loved one was not expected to survive, what would you do if faced with the decision of life supports?

6. After reading this personal statement, would you consider rehabilitation at any cost?

7. What would your response be if you and your family made every effort possible to "normalized" your brain injured family member yet they remained at a two-year-old's level of functioning?

8. Define and discuss quality of life.

9. What did Michael mean when he stated, "Head injury has no norm."

10. How can people learn to adapt to change like Laura and Michael did and are doing?

(SET 1)

CURING TRAUMATIC BRAIN INJURY

Perspective: What if an experimental drug was discovered that could eliminate the effect of a traumatic brain injury and restore a person to pre-injury levels of functioning? The cost is $25,000 per year.

Exploration:
1. Who should pay for the drug?
2. How should people be selected for treatment?
3. Should severity of injury be considered?
4. What if a person had a dual disability such as traumatic brain injury and severe mental illness?
5. Should a company be limited in the amount of money it could charge for such a drug?

(SET 2)

HOW LONG? HOW OLD?

Perspective: The reality of a severe head trauma may last months or years of a life time. This long-term perspective often can influence the process of making decisions and living with the consequences.

Exploration:
1. How long should a 10-year-old child be kept in a coma management unit?
    - a 38-year-old person
    - a 78-year-old person
2. What factors must be considered in making these decisions?
3. What does "forever" mean to families who are responsible for the emotional and financial well-being of a family member with a head injury?
4. How long should parents be responsible for a child?
5. How long should children be responsible for parents?
6. Should families be required to pay for medical and rehabilitation services if gains are not made?
7. Should long-term care facilities be required to keep a patient after funds are exhausted?

(SET 3)

IS THE PERSON WITH A HEAD INJURY MORE IMPORTANT THAN THE FAMILY?

Perspective: The occurrence of a severe disability in general and a head injury in particular often focuses all of the family's emotional resources on the person who has sustained the injury. Often this focusing is essential to contain the fall-out from the injury as well as to stabilize the total family system. However, in order for families to realign their goals and to establish a different balance in their lives, they must make a transition that considers the individual needs of family members, the total needs of the family and the emerging, changing needs of the family member challenged by a head injury.

Exploration:
1. In coping with the demands of a head injury in your family, how did/would you allocate emotional resources?
2. Is it ever possible to regain balance in the family following a head injury?
3. How long is a long time?
4. If you had a severely disabled child, a parent with Alzheimer's Disease, and a brain-injured spouse, how would you allocate your emotional resources?

(SET 4)

WHO SHOULD PAY FOR THE CARE OF A PERSON WITH A HEAD INJURY?

Perspective: In addition to the emotional and physical complexity surrounding head injury, families must also deal with complex financial realities.

If insurance is limited or non-existent or if large settlements are not viable, families are often forced to turn to other sources of support which are limited in scope and impact. At this point, families are forced to re-evaluate the situation and are often faced with very difficult choices. Often the choices are not who should pay, but who can pay, who wants to pay, and who is willing to help.

Exploration:
1. If you were in need of significant financial assistance from your family, would they respond? Why/why not?
2. Would you be available on a long-term basis to provide maximum financial assistance for a member of your family who had a head injury, spinal cord injury, AIDS, Alzheimer's Disease?

SET 5

MY FAMILY AND HEAD TRAUMA: WHERE DO WE STAND?

1. List five ways your family could be additive to the care of a family member with head injury.
2. If you had a head injury, would you want <u>your</u> family involved in your care. Why or why not?
3. What would be the most difficult aspect of family involvement for you?
4. What has been, is, or would be most difficult for your family in caring for a child who has a brain injury?
5. List the characteristics of your family which help in the care of a loved one.
6. What are the characteristics of your family which hinder the care giving process?
7. Do you feel that you are fully functioning in your own life so that you are a role model for other family members?
8. Would this change if you had a head injury?
9. Which family member would "understand" if you had a head injury? If you had AIDS?
10. Who would not be able to understand? Why?
11. Who in your family would be least able to cope with or adapt to illness? To head injury?
12. Can head injury be prevented?
13. If head injury can be prevented, why does it occur?
14. Would you be in favor of placing a limit on financial awards in head injury cases?
15. Should lawyers be limited to a 6% "commission" on all personal injury cases?
16. What is your position on sharing large awards with persons who were injured by an uninsured motorist who had no financial resources?
17. What are the benefits of a five million dollar settlement in a head injury case?
18. What are the liabilities of a five million dollar settlement for the injured person and their family?
19. Does the state have the right to mandate the use of seat belts and motorcycle helmets? If a person is head injured and not wearing them, should their insurance be reduced?
20. Write a question that has not been asked, that would be most important and relevant to your family's adaptation, coping, and survival of the head injury experience.

2

IMPACT OF HEAD INJURY ON THE PERSON

2

IMPACT OF HEAD INJURY
ON THE PERSON

A head injury can be as damaging to the personality as it is to the body. In fact, head injury is quite different from most other conditions that cause dependency because injury to the brain is often more pervasive in its effects than other conditions. Frequently there are limitations in mobility, cognitive ability, emotional stability, and other functional capacities (Anderson & Parente, 1985; Bergland & Thomas, 1991; DeJong, Batavia & Williams, 1990; Varney & Menefee, 1993). The effects of brain injury, such as difficulties with self-awareness, self-regulation, fluency of expression of thoughts and feelings, and inhibitions of emotions, can persist beyond the recovery period, and often result in long term personality changes and could affect the ability to function in relationships (Armstrong, 1991; Kaplan, 1993; Zeigler, 1987). Lezak (1986) believes that many persons with head injury have limited awareness of how much they have changed, and their greatest handicaps flow from impaired capacities for control, regulation, and adaptation of complex behavior.

The interactions of these limitations make the task of effectively working with persons challenged by head injury most difficult without first understanding the complex psychosocial problems related to the total head injury experience. The individual with head injury is usually attempting to manage the various emotional and cognitive changes, and while doing so creates other changes in one's family, and even creates a new meaning for family life (Riegel, 1976). If a person is continually angry about their limitations, for example, then frequently the anger will be projected onto others, creating an atmosphere of tension and anxiety. A head-injured family member who refuses to participate in proscribed therapies, claiming that "I don't have a problem with that," will cause frustration and disappointment within the family. The lingering presence of these emotions can inhibit the family from assisting their family member with head injury to achieve stabilizing rehabilitation goals. Optimum intervention, treatment and rehabilitation require, consequently, not only sound medical information, but also an awareness of the effects of the head trauma on the person with the injury and on the family lifestyle (Kerr, 1977; Livneh & Sherwood, 1991; Vash, 1981). This chapter will focus on the consequences of head injury on the person who has experienced the trauma.

SOME DETERMINANTS OF A PERSON'S REACTION TO A HEAD INJURY

Brain injury can be caused by a number of physical problems: trauma, anoxia, ruptured aneurysm, or brain abscess. Only in recent years have many persons been surviving the initial medical events which produce residual brain damage (Zeigler, 1987). This increased survival rate has facilitated the emergence of new treatment approaches, many of which emphasize the productive functioning of the total person after the injury itself. An understanding of emotional factors can play a key role in this functioning, but basic to this awareness is a knowledge of why the person with head injury is reacting in such a way. To be noted, however, is that such reactions are not static, but are more developmental. In other words, an individual with head injury may show specific reactions because of certain stages in the recovery and/or rehabilitation process. Soon after discharge from in-hospital rehabilitation care, for example, a person may display enthusiastic hope for complete recovery, and denial of any long-term limitations. In another phase of recovery beginning after six months, the individual may act irresponsibly, irritably, and be self-centered. At a later time, such as fifteen months or after hospitalization, the person may have become a difficult, childlike dependent family member (Lezak, 1986). As the expectation of full recovery by a person with severe impairment becomes less and less realistic over time, then a specific emotion, or a combination of emotions, may dominate this individual's behavior, such as depression, performance anxiety, defensiveness, and confusion. A lingering hope may later give way to temper outbursts with the gradual acknowledgment that certain head injury effects probably will be permanent. Yet besides specific recovery stages there are other determinants to a person's reaction to a head injury, some of which are:

1. **The personality makeup of the individual before head injury.** If a person is accustomed to being dependent on others for most daily needs, and has always been reluctant to show initiative or independent behavior, then that person may react to a head injury by becoming even more dependent than before trauma onset. If a person views himself/herself exclusively as a vigorous, sexually active, and physically strong individual, a head injury may cause heightened feelings of

depression and even despair. Other factors included in one's personality make-up prior to head injury are self-esteem, motivation, emotional needs, and vulnerability. Also, if before the onset of injury an individual has experienced many losses or severe illness, or has academically and socially achieved only with the greatest effort, or has had other physical or mental handicaps prior to the injury, or there is the presence of other serious illnesses in the family, especially another person who has had a head injury, then the individual with the current head trauma might be quite vulnerable to depression, and to choosing poor coping strategies (Christ & Adams, 1984). At the same time, these previous experiences might have assisted the person to learn more positive ways to adapt to this new loss. If, pre-injury, an individual had the continued satisfaction of competence in handling many life tasks, and one's emotional needs have generally been achieved, then gradually feelings of adequacy may return during post-trauma. However, due to depletion of resources, coping with a prior crisis does not mean that the person can deal with a new and unique experience such as head injury.

2. **Body image and related factors.** These include the type of symptoms, namely, whether they are disabling or in a body region that carries special importance, whether the head injury is closed or open, and the severity of the injury (Livingston & Brooks, 1988). For example, since a head injury may effect memory, this could be uniquely devastating to a lawyer. Similarly, if an athlete has the motoric ability affected, it could mean loss of career as well as personal identity. An open head injury may leave disfigurement which in turn may stimulate negative attitudes toward the person.

3. **The person's previous satisfaction with selected activities.** Though a head injury frequently causes decreased memory, if a person can recall during post-injury those satisfactions with paid employment or a leisure, marital, or household activity, these memories can provide a sense of satisfaction which, in turn, can stimulate hope and optimism during the recovery period. The depression which is such a lingering emotion with many persons who have a head injury can often be minimized with these moments of recall and the temporary conviction that such satisfactions may be regained. But the real loss consequent to head injury is that the pervading limitations resulting from the injury may preclude a person from maintaining a job and/or selected activities and thus necessitate learning new skills. Such a learning process may be a unique challenge for this population.

4. **Presence or absence of therapeutic intervention.** Appropriate early intervention could help someone to focus more on the residual assets than the limitations of head injury, and this perspective could help to minimize a lingering depression, as well as facilitate an aggressive attitude of coping rather than wishing head injury did not exist. It is not only the process of early intervention, moreover, which can make a difference in a person's emotional reaction. The attitudes of health professionals when providing treatment and/or rehabilitation can also have a decided impact on an individual. A physician or nurse who may only emphasize to the person what one cannot do instead of stressing the individual's residual capabilities may be almost inadvertently undermining the person's hope.

5. **Familial and societal reactions to head injury.** Family members can have a profound influence on how an individual will react to his/her head injury. Because of a head injury, roles within the family system are quickly and often permanently changed (Zeigler, 1989). Economic and relationship changes also occur, as well as the family changes resulting from dealing with unpredictable behavior. Issues of blame, consequently, often surface in the family system, and when the person with a head injury perceives these changes, guilt feelings accompanied by frustration and depression are frequently developed by this individual. A person with head injury also faces familial inconsistency, social injustice, and mixed attitudes from the family. Stereotypical ideas about head injury and unrealistic or negative expectations from family members concerning performance in the home all represent a challenge to the person with head injury and can foster feelings of inadequacy.

6. **Religion and philosophy of life.** For varied reasons, a person may feel that head injury is a punishment for past sins or believe that the acceptance of loss associated with head injury is an opportunity to meet a physical, as well as a spiritual challenge. Drawing from spiritual resources may alleviate feelings of anguish caused by head injury and may encourage hope. This hope may facilitate a more optimistic attitude which focuses on this life as a transition to the next.

7. **The life stage of the person.** People go through many life stages as they develop. The timing of head injury in the life cycle is particularly important. Most head injuries occur to individuals in the prime of life, a period in one's life when certain interpersonal and occupational tasks should be accomplished. Often someone has just begun a new career when the head trauma occurs. When the injury occurs at a time when there are great expectations, the emotional reaction could be more severe. For

example, a 21-year-old, unmarried man or woman living with one's parents may experience a head injury just at a time when college graduation or a significant job promotion is approaching. The injury precipitates a disruption in life plans, and the awareness of the disruption often facilitates depression and inappropriate behavioral outbursts.

8. **Ability to live with uncertainty and ambiguity.** Though denial of one's limitations caused by a head injury is a frequently recognized characteristic of individuals with head trauma, the different unpredictable cognitive, physical, and emotional aspects of head injury during the indefinite post-trauma period can be quite troubling to an individual. It may be a long time before there is symptom stability, and for individuals who are accustomed to having a measure of control over many life events, such as health, career, and family life, living with the unknown and episodic occurrence of symptoms may bring continued anxiety, irritability, and impatience.

9. **Specific location of the brain injury/lesion.** Healthy emotion, reasoning, and goal exploration are dependent on frontal lobe connections with the limbic system, and "emotional reaction is a collaboration between the left and right, superior and inferior areas of the frontal lobe, each which stimulates and inhibits positive and negative emotions." (Armstrong, 1991, p.17). Also, depression characterized by anxiety, fear, and sometimes agitated, hostile, or aggressive behavior can occur in right hemisphere dysfunction, while depression characterized by sadness, lethargy, and perserverative feelings can occur with left hemisphere dysfunction (Von Knorring, 1983).

EMOTIONAL REACTION TO HEAD INJURY

The uniqueness of each head injury, with its varied sequelae that causes a wide variety of cognitive, behavioral, physical, and emotional problems, presents a challenge in understanding the person's response to a head injury experience (O'Hara, 1988). Each emotional reaction will be unique, and the response will be influenced by a selective configuration of determinants. For one person, the emotional response may be greatly determined by such factors as family expectations, pre-trauma job experience, and the extent of damage to brain functions. For another, a person's reaction may be influenced by religion, early health care intervention, and one's developmental life stage.

Apart from the uniqueness of individual reactions there are certain themes that are evident across the lives of individuals recovering from a head injury. They are:

1. **Denial of the implications of the trauma.** Denial may include minimization of any personal threat, existence of negative emotion, loss of cognitive and/or physical abilities or the possibility that one will not completely recover. Denial with the person experiencing the effects of head injury may take the forms of denying past abilities or current limitations, pushing oneself too hard, and an unwillingness to give up control, identity, and value in the eyes of self and others (Armstrong, 1991). Deaton (1986) reports that denying past abilities may result in avoidance of grief, failure to participate in rehabilitation, and lack of motivation. Acting as though present status is identical to pre-injury status may also result in a failure to remediate deficits and alienation of family and friends. Deaton further explains that pushing oneself too hard can cause physical injuries and depression.

   Denial can also serve an adaptive purpose, for it can allow the individual to maintain a sense of self-esteem, reduce stress, and possibly generate encouragement and hope. Because of denial, the person with a brain injury can control, in so far as the individual has the capacity to do so, his/her perception of the trauma and one's emotional reaction to it (Matt, Sementilli, & Burish, 1988). All in all, however, although denial may reduce immediate distress, it frequently has a detrimental long-term effect (Watson, Green, Blake, & Schrapnell, 1984). If a person does not finally acknowledge the limitations caused by the head injury, then the recovery process may be considerably slowed down, and little remediation of deficits can occur.

2. **Grieving over perceived losses.** For those persons with head injury, grief is a profound sadness or sorrow due to the significant changes or reduction in such life areas as health, independence, sense of control over life, established roles inside the home, sexuality, familiar daily routine, and means of productivity. Importantly, grief is so many little dyings along the way of recovery and/or possible adjustment, and these little deaths continue to occur as the individual realizes that selected life functions may not be restored and one has to come to terms with the eventual possibility of little return to pre-injury capacities (Lewis, 1983). The grieving may be further characterized by the persistent desire for recovery of lost abilities, and the desire to express negative affect because of many losses but perhaps being unable to do so (Brown, 1990). The grief is often accompanied by feelings of anger and helplessness, with anger often directed toward others.

3. **Depression.** With the person's realization that he/she has limited control over one's life, and it is not within one's power to decide the future, then a depression is usually experienced.

In this kind of depression, feelings of anger, loneliness, frustration, isolation, and disappointment are associated more or less directly with the head injury trauma, and these feelings are almost expected after a disabling loss. The depression is part of the grieving process, and in this depression, the individual recovering from a head injury will experience, bit by bit, the impact of the varied losses upon his/her life. It is during this kind of depression that the person will express the anger, indeed the rage, that is every person's response to the anxiety associated with threats to oneself (Quigley, 1976).

4.   **Guilt.** Guilt is better understood in the context of interpersonal relationships. For example, family members may often express to the person with a head injury their beliefs about why the trauma occurred, such as not wearing a seat-belt or a motorcycle helmet. This blaming type of communication often results for the individual in feelings of inadequacy, shame, sadness, agitation, self-condemnation, and anger. It may be extremely difficult for the family and significant others to accept the reality of what has happened, and they consequently deal with their feelings by blaming the person with head trauma for all the changes.

5.   **Coping styles.** Individuals with a head injury will adapt selected coping mechanisms that represent strategies for dealing with the perceived losses. Denial is a popular coping style among these persons, but coping may also include a) displacement—anger over what one has lost may be displaced to relatives, friends, or others, b) regression—the individual reverts to past methods of gaining gratification, as, for example, when one formerly self-reliant becomes extremely dependent, and c) intellectualization, namely, when a person, especially if one is older when the head injury occurs, believes that, "I have lived a full life ... it could have been much worse ... perhaps I now will become a better person" (Brown, 1990).

Coping styles include the varied modes of dealing with the challenges ranging from pain, perceived losses, an uncertain future, redirection of goals, and relationship changes. These coping styles, whether they are more problem-focused, such as seeking information and support, or emotion-focused, such as releasing one's anger or accepting the situation with resignation, are constantly changing cognitive and behavioral efforts to manage specific external and internal demands that are viewed as taxing the resources of the person with an illness or disability (Matt, Sementille, & Burish, 1988). Many coping strategies are really palliative, such as problem-focused and denial that allow an individual to maintain self-esteem.

6. **Acceptance.** A recognition of limitations may eventually facilitate an appropriate life adjustment that includes gaining a new
perspective on living. The individual with head injury may begin
to be able to see that one's experience does not depend totally on
what has been lost and that one may eventually be able to handle
even a greatly altered life (Quigley, 1976). This acceptance is the
mental decision to live with the realities, the deeply ambivalent
feelings, and the new mode of living. New satisfactions or
capacities replace, when it is possible, those which have been lost
and old relationships are renegotiated based on new realities;
some will be given up and new ones will be formed. It is a gradual
process of redefining the self through new interactions based on
things as they now are (Quigley, 1976).

Integral to an understanding of a person's reaction to serious
head injury is attention to the re-socialization process that should
occur after the in-hospital phase of head injury treatment. Cogswell
(1968) has written about the re-socialization process with persons
who have a spinal cord injury. Often a similar re-socialization may
occur with persons who are brain-injured, namely, during outpatient treatment the individual will be cautious in the selection of
social opportunities, and when possible, carefully choose settings
that one has frequently used, and only associate with friends that the
person has had for a long period of time. Because one eventually
realizes the extent of physical, cognitive, and emotional limitations,
and goes through a period of re-adjustment of one's perception of
self-confidence, remaining abilities, and realistic opportunities, the
person with a head injury may become cautious about involvement
in any new life plans, associations, or even career opportunities.
Such cautiousness is a reflection of feelings of vulnerability and
"being different" that individuals with head injury will at some time
experience. On the other hand, a consequence of head injury could
be a very different reaction and the person could replace caution with
impulsiveness.

CONCLUSION

With an understanding of the complexity of head injury, both the
family and the health professional is better able to approach head
injury from a perspective based on hope tempered by reality. From
this frame of reference, effective interventions can be designed that
may help the person and their family to live more adaptively with the
realities of head injury as well as the other challenges of life and
living. The following personal statement, "Homecoming of a Brain-
injured Veteran," by Paul Murphy, presents the impact of head
injury on a person over a 25-year period. It is a sensitive journey
through loss, trauma, fulfillment, attainment, and validates that
there can be life after a head injury.

Personal Statement

HOMECOMING OF A BRAIN INJURED VETERAN
by Paul Murphy

In 1967, my family was going through a transition. My parents were contemplating a separation, my older brother had recently married, one of my sisters was leaving for nursing school, the other was just beginning high school, and I was entering the marines. The roles of my family were definitely changing and the family was facing a stressful time. It appeared that the family as I knew it was ending. It was apparent we would no longer be the same. My mother said with everyone leaving our house was too big to manage by herself, and moved into a small two bedroom apartment with my younger sister. The day before I left for boot camp I helped them settle into their new home. We all were starting over with new lives, new fears, new dreams, and new independence.

I could not wait to be on my own, because for the first time in my life I would be on my own. Little did I realize the military afforded very little independence. My independence was limited, but to a seventeen year-old, it was relished. However, that new independence was short lived. Halfway through my tour in Vietnam, I sustained a serious head wound that changed not only my life, but the rest of my family's.

My home address was my mother's apartment complex, so she was the first to hear of my injury. Through various sources I learned of the events that took place in my absence. My mother was very close with her neighbors and proudly told them all of her son, the Marine, serving in Vietnam. Whenever the postman came they would yell, "Gert, he's here!" and my mother checked the mailbox for a letter from me. One morning in 1968, a Marine officer and a Staff Sergeant showed up at the apartment complex, all who noticed were anxious with curiosity. This was a bad omen. The telegram they delivered said, "I had been seriously injured in hostile combat and sustained a head wound, that the prognosis was poor, and upcoming telegrams would keep them advised of any change." My mother was alone when the startling news was delivered and her reaction was that of shock and fear. Shock, that I was injured and fear that I could still die from my injury. The information in the telegram was minimal and the extent of my injury was not known. She would have to wait for the next telegram for information on any further progress.

The vagueness of the information about my injury brought about questions that would go unanswered for some time, which made the wait tormenting. Daily, my family asked the same questions. How injured was I? Would I live, and if I did live, would I be able to function? Foremost in my mothers mind was that I had a head injury. My mother's experiences with head injured victims was during World War II where most injuries to the head involved blindness. Telegrams began to arrive everyday and stated my condition was slowly improving, but there was still little mention of the actual extent of the injury. Telegrams reassured that my prognosis was improving, but questions as to how I would live as a blind person became the focus of my mother's concern, just not knowing was upsetting. She blamed herself for my being injured and was laden with guilt, because she felt it was her signature that allowed me to enter the Marine Corps in the first place.

Every little bit of information that was received helped lessen the burden my family was carrying and prepared them somewhat for my return, but they were still unsure what to expect. Due to the extent of my injury, I was unable to be transported to the United States for two months. This prolonged time furthered the agony and fears my family had. By being left in the dark about my injury, my family grew uneasy and constant feelings of hopelessness existed. A Red Cross nurse wrote a personal letter for me, but I was unaware of its ramifications. While the personal letter let my family know exactly how I was feeling, because I did not write it, it affirmed the notion my mother had, that I was blind. She went about rearranging her tiny apartment making it more maneuverable for a blind individual. It was assumed by the family that I would be living with my mother when I returned and that she would care for me. My mother was fearful of the severity of my injury and unsure whether she alone could handle caring for me by herself. Other members of the family offered support, but they did not live at home and it appeared that she would be carrying for me by herself.

When I finally returned to the States I was placed in Chelsea Naval Hospital. I remember my first day back in Massachusetts laying there on a crowded neurology ward. It wasn't long ago that I was on a train headed to Boot Camp in South Carolina. I was filled with the feelings of anticipation and excitement about the new life ahead of me. Now I was filled with sad feelings knowing that adventure was over and fearful of what the future held. My loss had been more than physical, I also had lost my family. I did not know who would be there for me.

The day my mother and brother visited me I was asleep. They were shocked to see me as an emaciated, shell of what I used to be. They were relieved to see that I was not blind, but were upset upon discovering my disability. Fragmentations from a mortar round had penetrated my skull and I was paralyzed on my right side; which was the reason for the Red Cross nurse writing my letter. According to the doctors, my damage was so severe that the chances of rejuvenation were very slim. I reassured them I could manage, but they fell over themselves trying to help. I had time to get familiar with my disability, but had difficulty dealing with their unnerving attempts to assist. I feared my future living a piteous existence with loved ones who felt they were helping me, but were only making it more difficult for me to be independent.

After six months at Chelsea Naval Hospital I went home, the only home available. My family had been in turmoil prior to me entering the military and I feared not having a permanent place to live when I got out of the hospital. I knew I could sleep at my mother's apartment on the couch when on leave, but now it was for an undetermined time. Home was my mother's tiny apartment, which was located on the third floor. I felt displaced, my old room and security was gone and I felt like an intruder. My disability afforded little mobility and the stairs became a barrier. I became a prisoner in a tiny two bedroom apartment. My mother had to deal with my complaining and progressive seizure disorder. I had daily grand mal seizures and very little medication care at that point. Nobody knew what to do, and we grew more tense in an already tense environment. My mother's only solace was weekly trips shopping with my sister-in-law. While I had a lot of moral support, no relief existed.

In spite of continuous tension between myself and my mother, I found her support be a valuable source of strength in dealing with my losses. She encouraged me to seek out new methods where I could express myself. At first I felt she was interfering, but realized if I couldn't change my body I'd change my mind. My younger sister also shared the apartment along with my mother and myself. She felt that her privacy was being imposed upon when I returned home. She had difficulty expressing herself to me and pretty much kept her distance. Being deaf and the baby of the family, she was used to getting all the attention, but when I returned that role changed. Having a disability she always was just a little different than the rest of the family, now I held that role of being different. She tried dealing with my difference, but it was both confusing and frightening to her. Like the rest of my family, she did not understand what was wrong with me. It took her a while to just get used to me being there invading her former privacy. I was a stranger to her; I was a stranger to my family.

Not long after I was home, my mother became a patient herself and had to deal with her own loss; she had a mastectomy. It was hard for me to show my depression when my mother was feeling so much pain with her loss. I felt compelled to help her after all the love and support she provided me in my losses. Her strength gave me strength. We provided each other with needed support over our losses and became closer than ever.

The roles of the family had changed drastically in three short years. My father held the family purse strings while I was in Vietnam and still managed to control them after I returned. Getting money for food and rent was painfully difficult. Money from the military and the Veterans Administration was long coming and nowhere in sight. It was a daily struggle. The difficulty drew my mother and myself together. My mother became less of a mother and more of a friend. We were like two wounded animals living in the same den. We were just scratching out an existence. My father continued to take the role he carved out for himself as a member of the family that was to be involved as little as possible. He did not live with us and was not affected by the daily traumas. He was not available to lighten the load and give either me or my mother a break from each other. My brother, however, became the significant male in the family for a short while. He became the muscles in the family doing all the difficult tasks a father would normally do, or we would do for ourselves. He became the main source of transportation and was depended upon for this by my mother and myself. When there was a difficult task he was called. This created friction between his wife and my mother. I also felt tension in our relationship. He felt obligated to do for my mother and me. I felt guilty he did so much. He unwittingly made me more aware of my disability.

My other sister was in nursing school and when she came home she became our source of constant medical questions. At first, she became overwhelmed and refused to answer anything, but after seeing me continuously having seizures was able to help come up with a good behavioral plan. Her skills and caring saved me from much pain. However, in the beginning it was difficult having her living at home and refusing to help. It took a while, but I was able to listen to my sister and I became a good consumer around my medical needs. I felt like an intruder with my disability, imposing upon my mother, brother, and sisters and at times they made me feel the part. It was difficult for every person involved with me and my change. The family spent a long fearful time not knowing if I would live or die or what condition I was in. They were happy to see me alive, but no longer knew who I was.

Conclusion

The roles of my family prior to the head injury were vague; we were all changing. After my head injury, more questions than answers were created. The questions of who would care for me seemed clear in the minds of some people–my mother would be the primary caregiver. No one ever asked her whether or not she wanted the job, or even if she was capable. The family members were thankful that I had not died. However, it was difficult having to live with a stranger who could be difficult to deal with.

The roles of my family became defined after I returned from Vietnam. While it was not their choice, they were forced to react to my disability. I know it was hard on my family when I came home. We could have used assistance in dealing with the trauma, but we received no professional help. Back in 1968, little was known about head injuries. They all were told I was lucky to be alive, and not to expect many changes.

Today, 25 years later, more information exists about brain injuries and the prevention of head injuries, but head injuries still happen. I have learned many lessons with my brain injuries. While no two brain injuries are the same, all brain-injured individuals require certain elements to mend. They need understanding, support, and time. Without any of these elements, no matter how severe the survivor's injuries are, they will have difficulty recovering.

My family provided me with understanding and support. It took time for me to mourn my wounds. While I was able to understand my losses, others may not be able to, due to the severity of their injury. What is important is that they are given the time for the insult to their brain to mend, and support throughout the process–support by family, friends, and the medical profession to help acknowledge the brain injured survivor's accomplishments, no matter how small. Most brain injury survivors hold onto yesterday and don't realize their losses. Usually "survivors" state they will get back to what they were before–chances are they never will. In their journey back they need realistic support as to their capabilities. It is a hard lesson to learn that you cannot do what you did before. Recovery for a brain injured person means living to the best of their potential.

DISCUSSION QUESTIONS ON THE PERSONAL STATEMENT "HOMECOMING OF A BRAIN INJURED VETERAN"

1. What would have made Paul's coping with his losses easier?

2. Is it "fair" that he had a head injury?

3. Could you have done as well as Paul if you were in his situation?

4. What happened to his mother? Was it "fair" that she became the sole caretaker?

5. Do you think he felt responsible for her illness?

6. What approaches would you use to have Paul's father become involved?

7. Is twenty-five years a long time to be challenged by the effects of a head injury?

8. What are the issues that should be attended to in the future?

9. How will Paul cope if he sustains another head injury?

10. Would Paul be prepared to cope better with a spinal cord injury because he has mastered and managed prior losses?

11. What kind of stress would be created if his wife became disabled?

12. If Paul had a child with a disability, how do you think he would cope?

13. How would you have assisted Paul's family to better understand and live with the effects of Paul's head injury?

14. What were the forces within Paul's support system that enabled him to excel and reach his goals?

15. What does living to the best of their potential mean for the person and the family living with a brain injury?

(SET 6)

HEAD TRAUMA AND THE FAMILY: HOW WOULD YOU LIKE TO BE TRAUMATICALLY HEAD INJURED LIKE ME?

Perspective: Imagine that you are 24 years old, living in a head injury rehabilitation facility and have been abandoned by your family. You are often told to control your anger and to get along better with your peers because you frequently become very hostile, and primarily express this during recreation periods. How should you feel? How would you feel?

Exploration: The point of this exercise is to explore some issues faced by a person living with a head injury and the need to appropriately express anger, frustration, distress and unhappiness. The challenge for the helping professional is to facilitate the expression of feeling, to reduce its negative consequence, and to create viable alternatives to counter-balance an often harsh reality.

1. Discuss the need to express anger, frustration, sadness, happiness, and hope.
2. How would you react to the partial loss of memory?
3. How would you try to get out of depression?
4. What are the implications of the loss of memory for you?
5. How would a traumatic brain injury impact your hopes, dreams and aspirations?
6. Would information on the severity of a head injury of a family member be helpful or harmful to you and your family?
7. Discuss how hope can be helpful and/or harmful.
8. Would a peer group counseling be helpful to you? Why? Why not?
9. What family resources do you have? Could you rely on them?
10. What would be the most difficult implications of traumatic brain injury for you? For a loved one?
11. Do you believe that miracles are possible even when there is limited optimism regarding physical improvements?
12. How would you spend your life if your future was altered by the occurrence of a head injury?
13. What would you do if your doctor told you to accept your injury in peace rather than seek out treatment or experimental drugs to "cure" your head injury?

14. How could your family be more helpful?
15. What do you feel you would need the most if you had severe head injury?

REFERENCES

Anderson, J., & Parente, F. (1985, July/August). Training family members to work with the head injured patient. *Cognitive Rehabilitation*, pp. 12-15.

Armstrong, C. (1991, April/May/June). Emotional changes following brain injury: Psychological and neurological components of depression, denial and anxiety. *Journal of Rehabilitation*, pp. 15-22.

Bergland, M. M., & Thomas, K. R. (1991). Psychosocial issues following severe head injury in adolescence: Individual and family perceptions. *Rehabilitation Counseling Bulletin, 35*(1), 5-22.

Brown, J. C. (1990). Loss and grief: An overview and guided imagery intervention model. *Journal of Mental Health Counseling, 12*(4), 434-445.

Christ, G., & Adams, M. A. (1984). Therapeutic strategies at psycho-social crisis points in the treatment of childhood cancer. In A. E. Christ & K. Flomenhaff (Eds.), *Childhood cancer: Impact on the family* (pp. 109-130). New York: Plenum.

Cogswell, B. E. (1968). Self-socialization: Re-adjustment of paraplegics in the community. *Journal of Rehabilitation, 34*, 11-13.

Deaton, A. V. (1986). Denial in the aftermath of traumatic head injury: Its manifestations, measurement, and treatment. *Rehabilitation Psychology, 31*(4), 231-140.

DeJong, G., Batavia, A. I., & Williams, J. W. (1990). Who is responsible for the lifelong well-being of a person with a head injury? *Journal of Head Trauma Rehabilitation, 5*(1), 9-22.

Kaplan, S. P. (1993). Five-year tracking of psychosocial changes in people with severe traumatic brain injury. *Rehabilitation Counseling Bulletin, 36*,(3), 151-159.

Kerr, N. (1977). Understanding the process of adjustment to disability. In J. Stubbins (Ed), *Psychosocial aspects of disability*. New York: Springer Publishing Co.

Lewis, K. (1983, July/Aug/Sept). Grief in chronic illness and disability. *Journal of Rehabilitation*, pp. 8-11.

Lezak, M. D. (1986). Psychological implications of traumatic brain damage for the patient's family. *Rehabilitation Psychology, 31*(4), 241-250.

Livingston, M. G., & Brooks, D. N. (1988). The burden on families of the brain injured: A review. *Journal of Head Trauma Rehabilitation, 3*(4), 6-15.

Livneh, H., & Sherwood, A. (1991). Application of personality theories and counseling strategies to clients with physical disabilities. *Journal of Counseling and Development, 69*, 525-538.

Matt, D. A., Sementilli, M. E., & Burish, T. G. (1988). Denial as a strategy for coping with cancer. *Journal of Mental Health Counseling, 10*(2), 136-144.

O'Hara, C. (1988, March/April). Emotional adjustment following minor head injury. *Cognitive Rehabilitation*, pp. 26-33.

Quigley, J. L. (1976). Understanding depression–helping with grief. *Rehabilitation Gazette, 19*, 2-6.

Riegel, K. (1976). The dialectics of human development. *American Psychologist, 31*, 689-700.

Varney, W. R., & Menefee, L. (1993). Psychosocial and executive deficits following closed head injury: Implications for orbital frontal cortex. *Journal Head Trauma Rehabilitation, 8*(1), 32-44.

Vash, C. L. (1981). *The psychology of disability*. New York: Springer Publishing Co.

Von Knorring, L. (1983). Inter-hemispheric EEG difference in affective disorders. In J. Flor-Henry & R. Gruzelier (Eds.), *Laterality and psychopathology*. New York: Elsevier Science Publishers.

Watson, M., Green, S., Blake, S., & Schrapnell, K. (1984). Reaction to a diagnosis of breast cancer: Relationship between denial, delay, and rates of psychological morbidity. *Cancer, 53*, 2008-2012.

Zeigler, E. A. (1987, Jan/Feb/March). Spouses of persons who are brain injured: Overlooked victims. *Journal of Rehabilitation*, pp. 50-53.

Zeigler, E. A. (1989, May/June). The importance of mutual support for spouses of head injury survivors. *Cognitive Rehabilitation*, pp. 34-37.

3

IMPACT OF HEAD INJURY
ON THE FAMILY

3

IMPACT OF HEAD INJURY
ON THE FAMILY

The head injury of a family member challenges the core values and resources of the family system. Not only must the family adapt to the emerging needs of persons with a head injury, but also it must continue to maintain a sense of unity by re-grouping its members, re-focussing its resources, and re-defining its functions. How the family reorganizes often depends upon its emotional response to the loss, stress, hope, and reality consequent to the head injury (Cavallo, Kay, & Ezrachi, 1992; Jacobs et al., 1986; McKindley & Hickox, 1988; Orsillo, S. M, McCaffrey, R. J., & Fisher, J. M., 1991; Rosenthal & Young, 1988; Williams & Kay, 1991; Zarski et al., 1988).

This chapter explores how family members react to the complexities of the head injury experience. Bringing these reactive patterns into sharper focus can enhance the understanding of the influences the family can have on the stabilization of the person with the head injury. Family members, for example, who deny the existence of a head injury or its complexity, are not going to effectively assist the patient during the treatment and rehabilitation process. At the same time, a family that has adapted to the implications and reality of head injury could be a constructive force in the person's life. However, since each family is unique and changing, so are the family reactions to the head injury of a family member.

DETERMINANTS OF FAMILY REACTION TO HEAD INJURY

There are many causes for why the family reacts as it does to illness and disability in general and head injury in particular. A knowledge of these factors not only may indicate why a family is reacting in a particular way, but it also suggests what may be done by health care professionals and other support systems to assist the family to adjust to a complex, demanding, and changing reality.

HOW THE FAMILY HAS DEALT WITH PREVIOUS CRISES

When a life crises represents a totally unfamiliar event, the family will usually display confusion and have a more difficult time focusing its resources. When previous crises have identified family resources, and helped to establish coping patterns, then the impact of the disability may be less devastating. Shock and a feeling of helplessness will still be present after the initial diagnosis, but these reactions may be managed more readily if the family has successfully managed other losses. A family that has weathered the experience of having a "breadwinner" out of work for many months because of a severe illness, for example, has had an opportunity to assess its resources as well as expand them. If another member of the family is diagnosed with a severe illness a few years later, the family will often adapt successfully if its resources were used effectively during the previous illness. If coping patterns have been effective in the past, then these will usually be adopted again in the new crisis. However, past success should be considered in the context of families not being able to deal with a new stressor, such as head injury, because their resources have not been replenished or new skills not developed or relevant to the unique aspects of a head injury.

THE MEANING HEAD INJURY HAS TO THE FAMILY

How the family understands head injury will depend on the kind of information that has been imparted to family members, when and how it was given, and the ability of family members to hear, understand and believe what is being said. Early and appropriate communication of information by health care professionals and significant others will generally diminish anxiety and allow the family to start working toward adjustment goals. If the family is in doubt about the nature of a head injury and its implications for the injured family member, this uncertainty will create continued family tension and inhibit the formulation of realistic goals. While information can be helpful, the complex long-term nature of a severe head injury can also create distress and precipitate a family crisis if family needs are in direct conflict with reality.

FAMILY INTERACTION

The family system which is nurturing, well structured, and has effective communication usually contains the potential to develop effective coping mechanisms. In contrast, in a family system where there are often indications of indecisiveness and contradictory types of behavior, family members will generally act in isolation from each other and have a difficult time reaching out to each other for mutual support. The head injury experience for this family will usually bring protracted periods of confusion and avoidance behavior in confronting the realistic implications of the head injury.

COPING RESOURCES/FAMILY CAPABILITIES

Coping resources include various emotional strengths that family members may possess to deal with head injury. Satisfying work activity, the support from extended family, the availability of necessary community resources, anticipation of planned activities, and self-help groups can be helpful in times of the continued stress associated with the head injury experience. Included in these resources are financial means and the ability of family members to use community agencies. A family that has financial protection and will not suffer severe economic hardship because of the head injury will theoretically cope much better than one for whom head injury represents a financial disaster. However, some financially secure families have become emotionally bankrupt while other "poorer" families have not only survived but have become emotionally rich. Given the astronomical costs associated with head injury care, few families can feel that they are completely financially secure and insulated from the long term issues related to lifetime care.

WHO IS ILL AND THE STATUS AND ROLE OF THE ILL FAMILY MEMBER WITH A HEAD INJURY

It may make more of a difference to the family if the wage earner or a child is seriously affected by head injury. For example, if the wife or husband is the major breadwinner and suddenly is brain injured, this could have a decided impact on overall family economic functioning. However, a head injury to a child can easily result in intense stress if the parents are unable to help each other during the acute stages of adjustment.

THE STAGE OF THE FAMILY LIFE CYCLE

Each family stage brings the necessity of accomplishing certain tasks (i.e., raising children or building financial security for the family). The presence of head injury has a unique impact on the family if the children had left home, and the parents were planning for their retirement years when suddenly they are looking at nursing homes or coma management facilities rather than retirement homes.

NATURE OF PRE-INJURY RELATIONSHIP TO INJURED PERSON

The family members' perception of their relationship to the person with head trauma is a critical component in how the family will adjust. If they perceive that the injured family member, prior to trauma onset, was an energetic contributor to family life, then their adjustment to the injury may be characterized by lingering feelings of loss, a reluctance to accept significant differences in the injured family member, and even a false hope that pre-injury functioning will be quickly restored. When family members believe that the person was a problem before the trauma, then this conviction will accompany their acceptance of cognitive and behavioral changes after the head injury event.

AVAILABLE SUPPORT SYSTEMS TO THE FAMILY

Support systems are defined as "continuing social aggregates (namely, continuing interactions with another individual, a network, a group, or an organization) that provide individuals with opportunities for feedback about themselves and for validation of their expectations about others ..." (Caplan, 1976, p.19). The availability of extended family, a support group, or a similar resource can make a difference in how a family copes with a head injury experience. These resources may provide respite care, nurturance, and feelings of acceptance to the family that convey the conviction that in spite of what has happened and perhaps the problem behavior of the family member, each family member is accepted as a worthwhile human being.

THE CULTURAL BACKGROUND OF THE FAMILY

The family's culture makes a difference in the member's adjustment to the disability. Afro-American families, for example, are organized around extended kinship networks which may include blood and non-related persons. Family roles, responsibilities, and functions are often interchanged among family members, a sharing which cuts across generations and gender roles (Carter & Cook, 1991). Among Latino families, there is variability among Latin Americans with regard to ethnicity, as in Puerto Rican, Cuban, and Mexican, as well as class differences. Traditional cultural values of fatalism, respect, spirituality, and personalism may be often reflected in the Latino adjustment to a disability event (Dillard, 1983). Within Asian families, moreover, transgenerational beliefs about coping with illness can be particularly important. The concept of obligation is also central in Asian cultures and families, and family obligations, such as providing care for a disabled family member, are communicated indirectly and by way of non-confrontational strategies (Carter & Cook, 1991). In other words, all families have distinctive cultural values and the impact of these values on the characteristics of disability and/or illness adjustment should be recognized.

THE ISSUES OF BLAME AND GUILT WITHIN FAMILIES BECAUSE OF HEAD INJURY

The factors of guilt and blame can be strong undercurrents for family members regardless of the cause of the injury. The perception of personal responsibility for the cause of a head injury can be a strong determinant in family member adaptation. If the person with a head injury takes responsibility for engaging in the behavior that caused the accident, such as alcohol consumption, or not wearing a seat belt, then other family members may adapt more easily to post-injury adjustment demands. Other family members may then feel less guilty. Even with this assumption of personal responsibility, family communications may be blame-laden or used as ammunition in family power struggles.

NATURE OF FAMILY STRESSORS

With head injury, physical and cognitive impairments of the person with the disability are usually perceived by family members as the most stressful. Included among family stressors are family finances, lack of respite care, limited living arrangements, continued anger in the family over undefined issues, and the special needs of the person with head injury.

If the health care professional understands the reasons why the family members are responding in a certain way to head injury, this awareness can form the basis for intervention. For example, when the health professional learns that the family has inadequate knowledge about head injury, and ascertains that the family members are emotionally receptive to further understanding and could profit from this communication, then intervention efforts might be directed mainly to imparting information which is based on facts but also conveys hope.

PATTERNS OF FAMILY REACTION TO CHRONIC ILLNESS

Historically, there have been contributions from researchers on family reactive patterns to long-term illness (Bray, 1977; Christopherson, 1962; Epperson, 1977; Giacquinta, 1977), these models are usually more appropriate when there are clear phases or steps in disability progression, and when the end result is more or less predictable. Armstrong (1991) believes that "family reactions to traumatic brain injury are likely to follow a developmental course, beginning with a response to acute stress which is reactive and crisis-oriented" (p. 10). Lezak (1986) and Romano (1974) developed models to explain a progression of family reactions, with Lezak emphasizing six stages of family adjustment to head injury, each characterized by distinct perceptions of the patient, expectations for recovery, and family reactions. These reactions range from thankfulness for the patient's survival, the family anticipating full recovery within the first year, and the family becoming confused and anxious as physical recovery begins to slow down, to family perceptions of the patient as difficult and dependent, a view accompanied by diminished expectations for improvement (Waaland & Kreutzer, 1988). Romano (1974) believed that families often have unrealistic expectations for recovery and rely heavily on denial, particularly during the early, post-injury period. She identified three common reactions:

(1) complete recovery was fantasized by family members; (2) denial causing physical impairments to be ignored or explained away; and (3) ignoring of inappropriate behaviors such as temper tantrums and deviant sexual behavior and the family's inability to establish limits.

When viewing caregivers' adaptation, these family reactive models to illness and/or disability may be less useful when the family situation is composed of a multitude of physical and/or emotional problems that have a much more indefinite course. As head injuries are so unique that no two individuals will exhibit exactly the same symptoms (Howell, 1978), so the reaction of family members will be different across families. Also, there is an episodic loss reaction by family members to head injury (Williams & Kay, 1990). The injured family member appears to be improving, family hopes are then increased, and then, unpredictably, there is a cognitive or physical setback, causing a renewed grief reaction among family members.

Within each family that is attempting to adjust to head injury, moreover, it is not unusual for husbands and wives to respond to the injury and subsequent losses in very different ways, and sibling responses may also be different. Grieving patterns may also be diametrically opposed, making it very difficult for family members to support as well as understand one another. Acceptance of the injury, consequently, may mean a realistic assessment and understanding of the significance and long-term effect of losses (Mitiguy, 1990). Mitiguy (1990) explains:

> Instead of an iron door, a thick but transparent curtain in the form of coma or disorientation descends between family members and the injured person. Their grief is suspended as they wait in hope for the curtain to lift and, later, for the patient to return to his former self. (pp.2-3)

Because of the uncertain course of head injury recovery, and the unique and diverse family reactions to the individual with head trauma, it is more appropriate to identify reactive themes, and then to suggest a model of family adaptation that captures the different ways that families may adjust to living with head injury.

THEMES

Shock: The onset of a traumatic brain event has a sudden, unexpected, and usually extensive effect on the life of family members. Feelings of helplessness, numbness, being overwhelmed, confusion, and perhaps even the temporary loss of self-control result from the initial event. At this time family members need to feel there is hope and that hospital personnel care about the patient.

Denial: With little information or understanding to what extent the patient will be impaired, family members may deny any implications of the trauma regarding permanent physical, emotional, or intellectual limitations. Denial may also take the form of insisting that the recovery will be complete, a divine intervention will occur, and minimizing any possible, future changes to family life. At this time, the denial may serve a positive purpose, namely, entertaining hopes may give family members the time and opportunity to identify and organize their coping resources.

Grief: Grief is a persistent feeling in families, an emotion resulting from not only the realities of family disruption but also caused by the loss of a family partner with whom family members had a mutual relationship and who cared about them and what was happening in their life. All of a sudden it becomes a one-way relationship and they miss the person who cared about them in a special way (Mitiguy, 1990). In fact, grief may be especially poignant for the injured person's spouse, since the essential loss of a partner is mourned, a mourning which is borne alone because society neither recognizes the grief nor provides the support and comfort that usually surrounds those bereaved by death (Zeigler, 1987). Family grief continues because family members remain in an uncertain state of waiting for full recovery but realizing that they may be dealing with the patient's impairments for the rest of their life.

Gradual Realization: As family members become aware that their injured family member is not going to be physically, emotionally, and/or intellectually the same as pre-trauma, issues of blame, guilt, anger, and depression emerge. Sibling responses may include withdrawal, hostility, sleeping problems, emotional outbursts, increased rebelliousness, and verbalized resentment (Mitiguy, 1990). During this time family members need to have questions answered honestly and to have explanations given in understandable terms (Mathis, 1984). They may also need to learn how to interact with physicians and other health personnel in order to gain the information they need and to combat their feelings of powerlessness.

Re-orientation: With the family's slow acknowledgment that the effects of the brain injury will be permanent, individual family members will gradually adjust their life to meet caregiving demands, role re-allocation tasks, and perhaps family finance changes. Although grieving can take on a chronic nature, many families do eventually work through feelings of denial, optimism, anger, and depression to a degree of adjustment. For some, this can take several years, and it can take very different amounts of time for members of the same family to come to some sense of resolution and acceptance. Yet many families start to educate themselves, seek out supports, assess problems, and plan for the future (Waaland & Kreutzer, 1988). During this period of re-orientation, fears about the patient's present and future preoccupy the stressed relatives (Armstrong, 1991).

This re-orientation of personal lives within the context of family life is very difficult for family members. Feelings of blame, anger, and resentment still linger, even accompanied both by a sense of relief that the injured family member did survive, and a conviction of hope that many previous functions of the person with head trauma will return. During this time of re-orientation, the family may attempt to re-integrate the injured person into family life, attempting to involve the individual in social activities and household tasks.

As the family engages in their adaptive tasks, and in their understanding that both anger and depression are parts of the grieving process, the physical, personal, social, familial, vocational and economic ramifications of the disability become apparent. Some families as a unit may welcome these changes and perceive living with the disability situation as a means for renewed family togeth- erness; other families may view the necessary changes as manage- able, and believe that their adjustment to the disability is an expression of their commitment and endurance and the family future is unalterably shaped by the head injury trauma; and still other families may perceive that the changes caused by the injury are catastrophic. The future of the person with head injury is hopeless, and that family life will now be characterized as troubled and lonely. Keydal (1991), in her study of families undergoing the adjustment process to a young adult, male member with head injury, refers to these three adaptive stages as success, survival, and submission. Yet it is not to be assumed that these family characteristics are represen- tative of the final stage in the family coping process to head injury. Adaptation to the head injury event is ongoing, and the family's long-term adjustment might be considerably altered as their percep- tions of living with the disability change (Keydel, 1991).

The different adaptive themes identified above can be illustrated in a sequential manner, assuming that there may be other reactions not identified that could be unique to families (Keydel, 1991).

Shock → Denial → Gradual Realization → Re-orientation → ↗ Success
Survival
↘ Submission

A recent study of developmental stage models (Rape, Bush, & Slavin, 1992) cautioned against a rigid adherence to stage models and indicated the need for more longitudinal research.

Integral to understanding the manner in which families react to the head injury situation is the awareness that family members will utilize different coping mechanisms as they attempt to adjust to living with the injury (Orsillo, McCaffrey, & Fisher, 1993). Varied coping strategies may be used for a period of time only to be replaced by other mechanisms. Coping strategies are employed to manage stressful demands, to ward off threats to family life, and perhaps even to change the situation. Families who appear to adapt well to the head injury utilize, with other resources, a more cognitive style of coping which expresses a sense of mastery in regard to their circumstances. Mastery can comprise a variety of skills, including skills for changing affective reactions to trying circumstances. Consequently, people who seem to adapt well to difficult circumstances are able to assign a meaning to their difficulties, as well as pinpoint the causes of their physical and emotional reactions to events.

With a cognitive style of coping, there are other ways to view the coping strategies of family members. Pearlin and Schooler (1978) have suggested the following three categories that are very relevant to illness, disability, and head injury:

1. Strategies to change the family situation (stress, anxiety, confusion, and avoidance by family members), caused by illness or disability. These can include seeking advice and information from knowledgeable persons, and tapping one's own individual strengths, such as communication skills and ability to identify valuable community resources.

2. Strategies to control, not change, family disruptions, anxieties, uncertainties for the future, and feelings of grief and loss. These strategies include positive comparisons formulated by family members ("We could be worse off..."), entertaining beliefs that the patient will improve somewhat or that support for caregiving responsibilities is available, utilizing tension reduction approaches, such as relaxation training or pursuing recreational activities, and accumulating knowledge.

3. Strategies to minimize personal discomforts caused by the reality of disability, such as stress, fear, frustration, disappointment, and future uncertainties. These strategies include ventilation, or talking with others about one's problems, distracting oneself with activities, stoically accepting the situation, and even wishful thinking, namely, imagining that someday the family situation will be better. For many family members prayers can also be an invaluable help to minimize feelings of grief and loss.

The coping strategies used by family members will generally depend on how the individual family member appraises the situation of living with head injury, and one's perception of the resources available. An individual makes a series of judgments concerning the potential effects of events on their emotional well-being. In other words, coping involves not only behavior but also varied thoughts on how best to deal with the situation.

The following personal statement, "Almost a Vegetable," by a survivor, mother, and father, explores the impact of a head injury from a survivor's, mother's, and father's perspective. During the difficult journey to stabilization and rehabilitation, each person drew upon their own unique resources and perceptions of the experience that had become part of their lives.

PERSONAL STATEMENT

ALMOST A VEGETABLE
by a Survivor, a Mother, and a Father

Changing from a fully functioning, young, athletic college student to a comatose, nonverbal invalid can take place in a matter of seconds. To recover may require years; some may never recover. For me, being alive today is a miracle. Following the motorcycle accident which resulted in a brain injury, my family was informed that it was unlikely that I would live. The following presentation is my perspective on my personal struggle to beat the odds. Not only was I able to win, but I was also able to rise above the physical and emotional strain placed on my life.

As a college student, I was at the point in my life of having everything going for me. I was happy as a university student, had a girlfriend, and was actively involved as a member of the track team. My preoccupations, at that time, centered around my independence, my future, and the variety of other joys and pleasures which were part of my life and that of my friends.

The summer prior to my senior year I was employed as a construction worker. To reduce the amount of time I would have to spend traveling to my home, I was living in a tent. It was a taste of the pioneer life, living in the outdoors, working and basically enjoying my sense of independence from my family. This need for independence and self-sufficiency had been an issue in the relationship with my parents and had caused some conflict between us. At this time I had no idea that I would soon become the most helpless, dependent person imaginable.

That summer, I was riding my motorcycle, enjoying the beauty of a summer's evening. My last recollection was that I was out of control. The next thing I remember was that it was November and I was in a hospital. Having no speech and being partially paralyzed, my life, at that time, was one of confusion, desperation, and challenge. I had a hard time putting the pieces together, but I somehow realized that I was hurting. I knew that I needed people to maintain my life supports since I would not do anything on my own. My decision at this time was if I am going to survive, I must draw people to me. I could not act up because I may drive them away.

What a difference to me at this time was the support given to me by my family and friends, who were always there. Their presence and encouragement made me want to make an effort to do as much for myself as others had hoped for me.

Being unable to speak since I came out of my coma, I was in a position of having to deal internally with the many issues that I was terrified and uncertain of, such as will I ever be able to speak, walk, or even approximate a semi-normal life. This is where the encouragement and input from the medical staff really made a difference for me. They conveyed a feeling of confidence and support that made me want to try even though I did not know how far I would be able to go. At this point in time, the personal relationships I had were just as important to me emotionally as the life supports were to me physically.

There was a critical turning point in my attitude when I began to attain some degree of independence. I became angry. I could not verbalize this anger, but it was there. It began to consume me. I went through the range of emotions, such as bitterness, hatred, disappointment, and fear. Here I was, 21 years old, a practical vegetable. How can I go on. I had a choice again: Either rise above it or die emotionally, physically, or both. I chose to live, to figuratively reach out and grasp whatever bit of life I could. I attribute this choice primarily to my experience as a member of the track team–having to be independent and reach inside myself to tap resources I did not think were there: To go the extra mile.

However, having made the choice, I had to still have the external motivation to go on. My nurses provided that. They were realistic, non-patronizing, attentive to me, and made me work hard. I saw them in the same light as a coach who was there primarily to help me win. At the same time, they gave me constant input, again being unable to verbalize, I was in need of the monitoring from the outside world. It is terrifying to think what would have happened to me if I was ignored.

I often wonder how many severely injured or ill people live in isolation and become stagnant because they are nonresponsive like I was. This is the thought I carry with me to this day, "How lucky I was that people did care". During my hospitalization, my brothers from the fraternity maintained a constant vigil. Their presence was an additional support to the family and medical personnel, especially during the difficult times when I was faced with major choices, such as, "Why try or why struggle".

As time passed, my attitudes of hopelessness, hatred, anger, and self-pity began to give way to hope and optimism. In retrospect I believe this can be attributed to the small gains that I was able to make. I could feel, begin to speak, and regained a variety of body controls. While great gains were not made, there was significant progress to have me appreciate the fact that I was moving, no matter how slowly.

A traumatizing thought for me was how would I have coped if I had to remain a semi-conscious vegetable for the rest of my life. When I considered the potential realities of what could have happened I suddenly become most appreciative.

As I reflect upon where I have been and where I am today–able to walk, talk with a slight impediment, and remember most things, I find myself aspiring to qualitative improvements in my life. I wish that my speech could continue to improve and that I could walk better, although if I had my choice, I would choose speaking clearer over walking better.

Interpersonally, I have many friends, but I am missing one important dimension and that is a girlfriend. Prior to the accident, I had a girlfriend–after it, I did not.

At this time, my major stumbling block is myself. I cannot see what any girl would see in me. Deep inside I guess I am hoping that I will make more gains prior to seeking out a relationship. My rationale is that the more improved I am, the better chance I have of not being rejected. However, I am aware enough to realize that the gains I make may not be tremendous and that I have to accept myself the way I am before another person could accept me. What I have going for me is my ability to place myself in situations where I can learn and experience new things. This is part of my personal rehabilitation effort to maximize my chances for success. I do not know how far I can go but I know that I will try.

Mother

My son has asked me to record some of my reaction to his accident, illness, hospitalization, and handicap. I look back over the past 2 1/2 years and I find my memory is fragmentary, surrealistic, and shrouded in fog. Therefore, I will present these thoughts as chronologically as I can but in a more or less stream-of-consciousness style; that is the way I remember them.

The call from the accident room of the Medical Center came at 6:40 p.m. on a Tuesday. The doctors reported that our son's condition was "grave" and that he had stopped breathing several times. I felt very calm as I reminded the doctor that he had been an associate of my late father, and that I wished everything to be done for my son. My husband and I rushed to the hospital prayerfully fearful.

Our son was in the critical care section, convulsing and surrounded by aides, doctors, nurses, tubes, machines, wires–and he was dirty. His father was sure he would live–I was sure that he would die.

The rest of the night was unreal–we learned as much as we could about the accident, we called our daughter, relatives, and physicians, signed papers, listened to reports–a 5% chance to live.

Most terrible of all was that there was nothing I could do but wait helplessly. For a month of coma, I waited. Through several infections, operations, x-rays, I waited. I asked, "Why?" There was no answer. I was terrified, and still there was so very little I could actively do.

School began, and I returned to work. This was a very great help to me–my mind was taken up and I was active. We all experienced a sort of "yo-yo" condition–way up with hope one day, down with despair on the next.

Friends, students, acquaintances, and relatives were extremely supportive. Finally, Ted came to. His eyes opened, he moved–not much but a little. He would blink twice for "no" and once for "yes". I really think I had hoped it would be like a soap opera–he would open his eyes, say, "Where am I?" and get up out of bed and come home. If I had ever known how very long it would be! He was moved from CCU to the neurological section of the hospital. This was somewhat traumatic for us all because the care was not so careful or so intensive. About this point, I really came to grips with the problem. I had stopped my why's and self-pity, swallowed some of my overwhelming pride, and accepted the fact that whatever happened, God's will, not mine, would prevail. At last I could cope.

Daily visits were the role. Ted still could not speak, but we discovered that he could read. Physical therapy was started; he could sit up with help. He looked awful–retarded–painfully thin like a survivor of Bergen-Belsen. Our physicians were optimistic and had stopped repeating, "The condition is stable; he's holding his own; his vital signs are good". How I hate those words! Tubes were removed one at a time–food, real food, was given. I was amused; Ted ate everything. He'd always been an exceedingly fussy eater, and I used to threaten, "Someday you'll be so hungry, you'll eat that!" Vindication #1!

On Thanksgiving Day, he came home to dinner. He still could not speak, had to be tied into the wheelchair so he'd not fall out, and a suprapubic catheter, and had to be fed. But he could smile; he could communicate (sort of), and oh, how he could eat! More chicken soup?

From that point on, he came home each Sunday and by Christmas he could talk–not always intelligibly, but talk. Astonishing to us all was Ted's personality change. He was cheerful, cooperative, and happy (this was very different from the sometimes surly, self-conscious, and somewhat withdrawn person we were used to). Somewhere along the line he'd learned to laugh at himself and to know he had to accept our help. Vindication #1; I'd told him that too!

In February, Ted was allowed to come home for a week. I was very apprehensive about this. He was pretty helpless–catheter still, not very mobile, had to be dressed. The one thing I'd never wanted to be was a nurse. I resent sick people, and mechanically (with tubes and such), I'm a klutz. However, I buoyed my sagging confidence by figuring I was as smart as some of the aides who'd been caring for him at the hospital (pride again). We both survived the experience. Ministering to a 6-foot-2 inch baby is different.

It was very difficult to return him to the hospital. But in another month he was home for good. We tried to keep everything as normal as possible. The only physical changes in the house were removing thresholds and one rug, and rearranging furniture for easier passage of the wheelchair.

Again, fortune smiled and sent us a young man who stayed with Ted two days of our working week, a girl one day, and our housekeeper the other two. These individuals were all involved in the rehabilitation process and were inventive therapists. I worried and tried to stave off any pitfalls (I am still too protective.). Hospital therapy was continued on an outpatient basis, and Ted worked very hard to recover. We all did.

A word here about the hospital–our son was at the Medical Center for seven months. He received excellent care, and we were supported by the interest and the involvement of the entire staff. Everyone from the lady who pushed the dinner cart to the senior physicians were exceedingly cooperative. I liked especially the honesty, humor, and realistic approach which everyone seemed to have. Questions were always answered. My only problem was in knowing what questions to ask. Our daughter took over at this point. She was preparing for two degrees, one in psychology and one in nursing. She knew what to question. Her sense of the ridiculous also smoothed some rough seas. When her brother started to talk (croak?) she spend the afternoon telling him jokes about people with speech impediments. He loved it! Whenever there was a new problem, his sister found the book where we could study and learn.

Ted's physical progress was coming. I hoped to keep his mind active and pushed him to plan and to return to school. I shuddered when he could not do things which seem so easy to us who have no physical handicaps, but I tried to be less fearful for him. We, his family, took him to restaurants, to stores, to sports events so that he'd be used to society. He moved from the wheelchair to crutches and, oh joy, in August, he participated as an attendant in a friend's wedding. Everyone was ecstatic.

He returned to college, commuting for the first semester and living at his fraternity the second. He graduated. Out of 1,600 black-clad seniors, he was the one with one crutch.

Now he walked, talked understandably, had a part-time job, and was accepted to graduate school. It was difficult for me to let him start off to the unfamiliar "big city" with so many problems. But I felt that he had to be independent and live his own life. He does.

How do I feel now? I have intense pride in his achievements and his hard work. I am greatly indebted to so many people for their interest and support. Most of all I'm grateful that he has been able to recover and that we as a family–my husband, my daughter, and I–have had the resources to help him. I hurt when he falls, but I try to accept it. We all try to be as realistic as possible about the future and to face it all with gratitude, with faith, and with humor. When people ask me, and they do, how does one survive a period such as this, I quote Pearl Buck, who had one of her suffering characters reply, "I really cannot face it, but I must".

Father

I was working in the garden when my wife came running out saying, "Teddy's had a motorcycle accident and it's bad." I went cold and thought, "Oh, my God, he's dead. Can Charlotte stand it?"

From then on I did what had to be done, driving cautiously to the emergency room, going to critical care, seeing Teddy mechanized and with blood on his face but not really marked. I don't remember my thoughts. I do recall thinking "He's not dead yet." I called people. Without being reminded, I'm not sure who beyond my sister-in-law.

I don't remember what I said. Teddy's sister and her friends arrived. We sat in the CCU waiting room waiting with others who were waiting as we were. It was a close community–we became close.

There were the crises. I prayed he would die rather than become a vegetable. I don't remember the point at which I knew he would not die. It wasn't many days after the accident. At that time, I came back to earth and realized what was and what might be. I cried.

From then on it was a treadmill on which I thought about the outcome as little as I could force myself to do. The details of the first six months or so are blurred. I probably prefer it that way.

As Teddy improved my biggest concern was, "How much are his intellectual and reasoning faculties damaged? And if they're not what dents will being crippled put in his psyche?"

My background as an engineer puts a lot of trust in absolutes. If this is done, that will result. Although I know what statistics are, the two-year limit on improvement weighed heavily. Would he improve to the point where he would see the future as promising?

At the present stage in his recovery, I'm sure he has answered the questions I had, and if no further physical improvement is made, he'll still be able to make his way. The fact that I see continuing improvement is added frosting on a cake that is already much larger than I dared hope.

DISCUSSION QUESTIONS ON THE PERSONAL STATEMENT "ALMOST A VEGETABLE"

1. How would your family respond if you were head injured while riding a motorcycle when they told you never to get on one?

2. What are the assets and liabilities of being strong-willed and determined not to be a "vegetable?"

3. How did Ted's parents' personalities and resources complement each other?

4. Why was the family able to respond in a unified manner?

5. How do you think they would have responded if Ted did not make the great gains that he did?

6. How could an "engineering perspective" as presented by Ted's father, be helpful or frustrating in coping with the complexities of head injury or any other disability?

7. Compare your families coping style, life values, and resources to Ted's family?

8. How would your family respond in this situation?

9. What would they need to cope and maintain their quality of life?

10. How do think this family would respond if the mother, father, or sister became disabled? Were brain injured?

SET 7

PRIME OF LIFE

Perspective: Head injury never occurs at a "convenient" time in a person's life. Having read the prior personal statement, try to imagine what your life would have been like if you experienced an injury when you were a young adult.

Exploration:
1. If you were as severely injured would your girlfriend or boyfriend remain with you?
2. Would you have preferred to be at home or away from home during your rehabilitation?
3. Would your family have responded in a similar or dissimilar manner?
4. What would you have needed to maintain a sense of control, independence and dignity?
5. Should people who do not wear helmets when riding a motorcycle be covered by insurance or eligible to sue if injured?
6. How would you respond if your son was brain injured as a result of a motorcycle accident, made great gains, and wanted to buy another motorcycle so he could feel normal again?
7. What is the responsibility and liability of a person who gives a ride to someone and they are head injured?
8. Do parents have the right to request that a severely brain injured child not be recuscitated? Brought to a hospital? If such a request is made and the child is given medical care over the objections of the parents, who should be responsible for the life long-care of the child?

REFERENCES

Armstrong, C. (1991, April/May/June). Emotional changes following brain injury: Psychological and neurological components of depression, denial, and anxiety. *Journal of Rehabilitation*, pp. 15-21.

Bray, G. P. (1977, March). Reactive patterns in families of the severely disabled. *Rehabilitation Counseling Bulletin*, pp. 236-239.

Caplan, E. (1976). The Family as a support system. In E. Caplan & M. Killilea (Eds.), *Support systems and mutual help* (pp.19-36). New York: Grune & Seratton.

Carter, R. T., & Cook, R. T. (1991). A culturally relevant perspective for understanding the career paths of visible racial/ethnic group people. Submitted for publication in Z. Leibowitz & D. Lea (Eds.), Adult Career Development. National Career Development Association.

Cavallo, M. M., Kay, T., & Ezrachi, O. (1992). Problems and changes after traumatic brain injury: Differing perceptions within and between families. *Brain Injury, 6*(4), 327-335.

Christopherson, V. (1962, February). The patient and family. *Rehabilitation Literature*, pp. 34-41.

Dillard, J. M. (1983). *Multi-cultural counseling*. Chicago: Nelson Hall.

Epperson, M. (1977). Families in sudden crisis. *Social Work in Health Care, 2-3*, 265-273.

Giacquinta, B. (1977, October). Helping families face the crisis of cancer. *American Journal of Nursing*, pp. 1585-1588.

Howell, C. (1978). Braindamage. In R.M. Godenson (Ed.), *Disability and rehabilitation handbook* (pp.284-295). New York: McGraw-Hill.

Jacobs, H. et al. (1986). Family reactions to persistent vegetative state. *Journal of Head Trauma Rehabilitation, 1*(1), 55-62.

Keydel, C. F. (1991). *An exploration of perception and coping behavior in family members living with a closed head injured relative.* Unpublished doctoral dissertation, University of Maryland, College of Education, College Park.

Lezak, M. D. (1986). Psychological implications of traumatic brain damage for the patient's family. *Rehabilitation Psychology, 31* (4), 241-250.

Mathis, M. (1984). Personal needs of family members of critically ill patients with and without acute brain injury. *Journal of Neurosurgical Nursing, 16*, 36-44.

McKinlay, W., & Hickox, A. (1988). How can families help in the rehabilitation of the head injured? *Journal of Head Trauma Rehabilitation, 3*(4), 64-72.

Mitiguy, J. S. (1990, Fall). Coping with survival. *Headlines*, p. 228.

Orsillo, S., McCaffrey, R. J., & Fisher, J. M. (1991). The impact of head injury on the family. The Journal of Head Injury, 2(4), 19-24.

Orsillo, S. M., McCaffrey, R. J., & Fisher, J. M. (1993). Siblings of head-injured individuals: A population at risk. *Journal of Head Trauma Rehabilitation, 8*(1), 102-115.

Pearlin, L. I., & Schooler, C. (1978). The structure of coping. *The Journal of Health and Human Behavior, 19*, 2-21.

Rape, R. N., Bush, J. P., & Slavin, L. A. (1992). Toward a conceptualization of the family's adaptation to a member's head injury: A critique of developmental stage models. *Rehabilitation Psychology, 37*(1), 3-22.

Romano, M. (1974). Family response to traumatic head injury. *Scandinavian Journal of Rehabilitation Medicine*, (6), 1-4.

Rosenthal, M. & Young, T. (1988). Effective family intervention after traumatic brain injury: Theory and practice. *Journal of Head Trauma Rehabilitation, 3*(4), 41-50.

Waaland, P. K., & Kreutzer, J. S. (1988). Family response to childhood traumatic brain injury. *Journal of Head Trauma Rehabilitation, 3* (4), 51-63.

Williams, J. M., & Kay, T. (1991). *Head injury: A family matter.* Baltimore: Paul H. Brookes Publishing Co.

Zarski, J. et al., (1988). Traumatic head injury: Dimensions of family responsivity. *Journal of Head Trauma Rehabilitation, 3*(4), 31-41.

Zeigler, E. A. (1987, Jan./Feb./March). Spouses of persons who are brain injured: Overlooked victims. Journal of Rehabilitation, pp. 50-53.

4

FAMILY CONSIDERATIONS IN ADJUSTMENT TO HEAD INJURY

4

Family Considerations In Adjustment To Head Injury

There are specific reasons why some individuals and families do not make more progress toward feasible adaptation goals. This chapter explores some causes of family maladaptation as well as successful adjustment to a head injury. In becoming aware of these reasons, families and health care professionals can better pursue mutual rehabilitation goals. For example, if the presence of chronic stress within the family inhibits any efforts to conceptualize, approximate, or reach goals, then steps could be taken to alleviate this stress by teaching and modeling familial survival skills appropriate to the situation rather than accepting stress as a necessary by-product of the head injury experience.

An understanding of the family influences that can affect the person with a head injury is essential for effective intervention. Head injury can produce recurrent crises within the family simply because of the multidimensionality of the effects of a head injury. When the diagnosis implies an ongoing uncertainty, often chronic stress occurs in the family. Following the initial shock of the injury, and often because of the temporary confusion among family members, family life can become uncertain and living with the effects of the head injury, an ongoing challenge. Adaptation will also be more difficult if there are other illnesses or stresses within the family that must be attended to in order to facilitate rehabilitation of the family member.

This chapter will identify the many family influences, comprising family strengths and family problems, which can shape family adjustment and their own management efforts to the head injury situation. It will also explain family adaptive and maladaptive patterns to head injury. An understanding of these patterns can offer insights into the most appropriate intervention approach.

FAMILY STRENGTHS

The identification of family strengths can pinpoint family resources, serve as reinforcements for family members, and indicate guidelines for intervention. From the authors' work with families, they have identified the following family strengths, each of which suggests to the professional a needed area for appraisal and a possible pathway for intervention.

THE ABILITY OF THE FAMILY TO LISTEN

Many families with a member who has a head injury are caught up with their own sense of loss and anxiety, especially during the early stages of health care intervention. But if family members have the ability, despite these emotions, to listen to each other and to the information provided by medical and related staff, then intervention planning may be implemented effectively.

SHARED, COMMON PERCEPTIONS OF REALITY WITHIN THE FAMILY

This family strength refers to a knowledge among family members of their own limitations, the physical and emotional resources to deal with a family change, and what the treatment and adjustment needs of the patient are. It includes an eventual acceptance of the reality of head injury, and many of its implications for family life. Though family members may still hold on to their denial of specific implications of the injury, such as an acknowledgment of permanent cognitive and physical changes, they are attending to management concerns and the performance of necessary family duties.

THE ABILITY OF FAMILY MEMBERS TO TAKE RESPONSIBILITY FOR DISABILITY-RELATED PROBLEMS

What this strength implies is the attitude that, "I can prevent family problems if I can take responsibility." This strength is illustrated by such questions as, "Since my child had an accident and is now head injured, what are the family needs that must be met for adequate family functioning?" Or, "Who is going to help me with some of the family chores, such as paying bills or attending to the treatment concerns of my child?"

The early assumption of selected family tasks may prevent later problems, such as neglect of the person, resentment among younger family members, and isolation of family members from each other because of a perceived lack of attention. In other words, this strength implies that family members confront the demands of the disability situation and begin to tackle the many issues that arise when living with a person who has a head injury or other disability.

THE ABILITY OF FAMILY MEMBERS TO USE NEGOTIATION IN FAMILY PROBLEM SOLVING

This family strength could be one that may have taken many years to develop and has been utilized many times before the occurrence of a disability or a head injury. It means that family members are willing to talk with each other about various options over a course of action, are able to compromise some of their own wishes, and are open to family-life suggestions from other family members. Though family members may react differently to head injury, when a decision is reached about what should be done, it represents an action that has collective input.

FAMILY MEMBERS' WILLINGNESS TO TAKE GOOD CARE OF THEMSELVES

This strength includes the family's ability to use well their leisure time, to relax and to seek a balance between family responsibilities, work, and recreation. It implies that family members have the conviction that they must, to survive living with a head injury experience, take appropriate care of themselves. Frequently, however, family members become guilty if they attempt to seek legitimate respites from caring efforts. The authors have heard often from a family member, "My work is 24 hours ... this is my mission in life." But when the family has periodic, legitimate outlets, a renewed source of vitality is available. In turn, this energy often becomes the stimulus for family members to be supportive for each other.

THE FAMILY'S ABILITY TO FOCUS ON THE PRESENT, RATHER THAN ON PAST EVENTS OR DISAPPOINTMENTS

Family members usually bring to a head injury experience much of their unfinished, emotional business. It might be a past regret, an unresolved anger, or a lingering resentment. Such emotions can get in the way of family togetherness. Anger often facilitates the isolation of family members from each other. Yet family members need to be encouraged to emphasize what is happening now; to use constructively the present opportunities in the home, on the job, and with friends; and not to dwell constantly on the past or on an uncertain future. It is difficult for family members to forget or to suppress negative emotions, but when they can it is another pathway to their helping each other in this disability situation.

THE ABILITY TO FAMILY MEMBERS TO PROVIDE REINFORCEMENTS TO EACH OTHER

Most families have a pattern of positive reinforcements that appear to make family life more satisfying. It may be spending some time playing with the children, or an hour of allowed private time, and outing together to a favorite restaurant, a meal cooked by a significant other, or physical and emotional love shared by the spouses. Whatever it may be, the onset of illness, disability, or a head injury does not have to eliminate completely such important critical forms of nurturance. Frequently, family members have to be encouraged to restore these satisfactions to each other which enrich the quality of family life.

THE ABILITY OF THE FAMILY MEMBERS TO DISCUSS THEIR CONCERNS

This strength can also be called "Family Expressiveness." It involves the family members' capabilities to talk to other family members, extended family, selected friends, and helping professionals about the impact of the disability experience on themselves, to share their disappointments, and perhaps even to tell health care workers that they are torn between compassion, guilt, anger and rage when taking care of and living with the person with a head injury.

THE ABILITY OF FAMILY MEMBERS TO PROVIDE AN ATMOSPHERE OF BELONGING

This strength means the family's willingness to convey to the person with a head injury that, "You are still an important member of our family." The authors' experience with families and disability (Power & Dell Orto, 1980; Power, Dell Orto, & Gibbons, 1988) has often suggested that, after the onset of a serious illness or a traumatic disability, family members may tend to become isolated and distanced from the person experiencing a disability. Family members may have difficulty adjusting to many disability manifestations, especially those associated with head injury. But if both the person and their family are going to adjust to the head injury experience, they must feel that they still "matter."

THE FAMILY PRESENCE OF EFFECTIVE TRANSGENERATIONAL COPING STRATEGIES

In discussing the relationship between behavior and coping, Rolland (1988) and Keydel (1991) have indicated that within families patterns of behavior emerge that express how family members may cope with an illness or disability event. Families bring their own history of managing an illness situation to the occurrence of head injury. If a family believes that eventually they can control the impact of the disability on family life, a sense of control that has been existent within the family for several generations, then definite coping patterns become apparent. If family members are accustomed to providing mutual support in a crisis situation, and this support is a learned, coping behavior that is integral to a family's history, then usually this form of coping will be utilized during adjustment efforts to a head injury.

SELECTED FAMILY PROBLEMS CAUSED BY THE HEAD INJURY

There are many family problems related to head injury that represent a possible influence on the adjustment of the person with head injury (e.g., chronic stress, poor interpersonal functioning, lack of information, negative sick role expectations, social isolation, a lingering grief, sexual concerns, and untimeliness of the injury). In concert, these problems can stress resources and challenge the family system.

CHRONIC STRESS

Jaffe (1978), identifies chronic stress as a "pathway by which family relationships contribute to illness" (p. 333). The presence of continued stress in the family can seriously hamper the clients' adjustment, motivation, and willingness to respond to intervention efforts. It also prevents a family from developing necessary coping mechanisms to deal with the ongoing demands associated with head injury. In a stressful family environment, the family is primarily attempting to survive. This is difficult to do when the stress is characterized by anxiety, fear, irritability, resentment, and hopelessness, all of which can prevent functional adaptation.

The origins of this stress are many, namely, the patient's emotional reaction to the injury, the possible abandonment behavior of family members, severe financial concerns, and the uncertainty generated by not knowing if the person will make meaningful rehabilitation gains. The following are examples of such situations: 1) A patient's anger over the debilitating effects of head injury which creates constant tension in the family. 2) Siblings who moved away from the home may cause stress because they did not want to become involved. 3) If head injury has brought to the family members new financial restrictions and the family is concerned about meeting their bills, or are even at the point of a major financial disaster. All of these are stressors which, if left unchecked, can be problematic and destabilizing to the family.

INADEQUATE INTERPERSONAL FUNCTIONING AMONG FAMILY MEMBERS

The family's level of functioning suggests how its members are able to adapt to head injury or utilize coping resources. The family that is continually disorganized and unable to provide for the emotional functioning of its members will find it too difficult to become focused and directed toward stabilization goals. Family members may find it difficult to communicate their needs because of emotional barriers. There also may be limited and conditional affection shown between family members, and blaming others may take over as a dominant communication style. In contrast a family that is able to provide support to its members, and can actively look for solutions to problems will frequently be able to meet the demands associated with head injury. However, both health care professionals as well as families must be aware of the enormity of the demands related to head injury and the need to view coping as a journey and not a destination.

LACK OF INFORMATION

Information refers to the understanding the family members have about head injury and the personal meaning of head injury to the survivor as well as the family. This knowledge includes the physical and emotional aspects of head injury, the rehabilitation potential, what extent each family member views the head injury as actually disabling and what it personally means to them, and an understanding of available resources. A frank revelation of these facts pertaining to head injury may cause shock, uncertainty, despair, resentment, as well as hope. When the families are given important and appropriate information about head injury at the time of onset they are given the opportunity to "work through" their feelings and set the stage for adaptation. They are also given the chance to appraise realistically the situation in order to make future plans based on reality of hope, support, and caring. A lack of relevant information can cause confusion and anxiety among family members. If the family is unaware of available resources, they can miss an opportunity to benefit from a potential support system.

The uncertainty about head injury generally causes apprehension and lingering fear of the unknown. It also inhibits the establishment of family plans that focus on future adjustment. After becoming aware of the characteristics of head injury, what complications may occur, and learning appropriate coping procedures, the family is better prepared to deal with ongoing and developing problems as well as develop proactive coping strategies.

NEGATIVE SICK ROLE EXPECTATIONS

Expectations related to head injury usually flow from the family understanding of the injury. For example, if the family perceives that head injury causes a person to be different and not just to act differently on occasion, they place the person and themselves in a difficult situation, believing that the person could do better if more effort was made. This attitude prevents the person from continuing appropriate family duties, and often encourages failure by encouraging unrealistic expectations.

However, when families are given information that emphasizes the individual's assets, family members begin to think more positively about the future since they want the person to continue to function as optimally as possible for as long as possible, given the reality that the person they knew has changed. This is the poignant point made in the classic book "The Humpty Dumpty Syndrome" by Janette Warrington (1981).

SOCIAL ISOLATION

Families frequently focus all their attention on the person with a head injury and neglect their own personal needs. Social opportunities that were part of family life may be put aside because of management issues, feelings of guilt, or the individual family member's perception that one is competent to assume caregiving responsibilities. This isolation gradually erodes the family member's energy to accomplish family tasks. Lack of respite opportunities may gradually heighten feelings of frustration and disappointment at the patient's lack of progress.

LINGERING GRIEF

With the return of the person with a head injury to the family, grief over the loss of function and "what might have been" is a constant companion to family life. Grief is an expected emotion following a trauma, but it can show itself in frequent, behavioral outbursts. These outbursts, may in turn stimulate confusion in the person with head injury and only add to family stress.

SEXUAL CONCERNS

Sexual concerns and behavior contribute to problems within the family and are frequently a source of stress. Unfortunately, most couples and families are hesitant to discuss sexual problems resulting from head injury. Many couples complain of excessive sexual demands from the head injury partner, or they feel that their spouse does not understand an apparent diminished sexual capacity. These complaints and perceptions generate a tension between the spouses that in turn causes them to become more easily irritated with other family members. In such an environment it is difficult for family members to be empathetic to a situation they may not be able to comprehend. Zeigler (1987) addresses the complexity of the issue in her article "Spouses of Person who are Brain-Injured: Overlooked Victims." This article focuses on the changes in behavior as well as the complex emotions of living in an altered relationship.

UNTIMELINESS OF INJURY

Most head injuries occur with males between 18-30 years old, a time in the family life cycle when many parents are looking forward to their own, diminished parental responsibilities and more freedom to pursue individual or mutual interests. The family disruption that is caused by head injury only increases when other family members perceive that future plans must be changed and even new caregiving role must be assumed. Anger, resentment, and disappointment are feelings that may be difficult to control because of the unwelcomed family transition.

MALADAPTIVE AND ADAPTIVE PATTERNS

Because of many negative influences from within and without the family, maladaptive patterns occur that can affect a person's adjustment. The family members can deny the reality of head injury to the extent that inclusive treatment considerations are ignored. They may attempt to eliminate head injury related problems by ignoring them. Also due to family dysfunction, the members may have to cope individually, leaving the person alone while they attempt to survive. The long term effects of head injury may eventually cause the spouses to divorce, or collapse physically and emotionally, although it is important to note that the head injury experience has enabled some families to become closer and more functional. Yet what is important for families and health professionals to understand are the causes of these maladaptive family reactions; to identify them is to become aware of what kind of intervention is needed. Rakel (1977) described five criteria that are relevant to a family's adjustment to disability and are applicable to head injury. They are:

1. Internal role consistency among family members. Each family member has a conception of what is expected, and this should be consistent with what other members expect.
2. Consistency of family roles and actual role performance.
3. Compatibility of family roles with community norms.
4. Meeting the psychological needs of family members.
5. The ability of the family to respond to change.

Duvall (1971) believes that families best able to undergo change during stressful situations and maintain family equilibrium show the following characteristics:

a. They approach problems in a unified manner as a family.
b. They have a nonmaterialistic orientation.
c. The husband and wife frequently share tasks.
d. They perceive the nature of the problem accurately.
e. They have a democratic orientation, with diffusion of leadership regarding problem-solving tasks.

Families that can adapt positively and are able to make good adjustments share other features, such as effective and constant communication, flexibility of family roles, tolerance for individuality, marital adjustment characterized by satisfaction, happiness, and stability, social participation of wives outside the home, and ability to support each member's self-esteem (Rakel, 1977).

CONCLUSION

The reality of head injury in a family can generate closer relationships among family members or it can fragment the family and create a state of disorganization and dysfunction. Early and ongoing intervention by health care professionals and other support systems is absolutely necessary because they can be effective catalysts for successful coping and eventual adjustment. However, health care professionals must be aware that all families bring a very complex and personal history to the head injury experience.

The following personal statement, "I'm Just Waiting for the Worse to Happen," reflects the agony, pain, sorrow, and frustration of a mother who is living with the ravages of a head injury, and just waiting for the worst to happen.

Personal Statement

... I'M JUST WAITING FOR THE WORST TO HAPPEN
(A Mother's Perspective)

I was 56 on my last birthday and I feel like I'm 90. There are days when I don't think I can last the day at my job as a public school custodian. I'm a separated white woman living in a city row house with a 28-year-old head injured son who acts like he's three. The kids in the elementary school where I work have more sense. You would think that he would have learned from his accident to be a responsible law abiding person but instead his behavior just gets worse every day. Not a day goes by that I don't expect the police to pick him up for something. I have two older sons who live out of the city. One is married and the other one is divorced. They can't stand to be around their brother so they don't come around much anymore. They think I should kick him out.

Two years ago he and another boy were high on some kind of drug and racing each other on their motorcycles. My son slammed into a telephone pole. He never wore a helmet. They say if he had had a helmet on, he probably would be okay today and can you believe that he says that if he could ride a motorcycle now, he still wouldn't wear a helmet. He can't ride one because of the paralysis on his right side. His paralysis doesn't keep him from doing lots of other irresponsible things. He is never home and the people he hangs around with are trash. They all drink and take drugs and none of them have good jobs. My son gets S.S.I. and that money is gone the minute he gets his hands on it. Then he wants to borrow from me.

He wasn't this bad before the accident. I never had to worry about him. At least he worked. He planned to some day work in the shipyard like his father. If he used drugs, it wasn't often and only if his friends talked him into it. He didn't have much ambition but I figured that once he got married, he'd work harder and start to save some money. He had a nice girlfriend. After the accident, when he came home from the Rehabilitation Center, she hung around for a little while but then she stopped coming. I think he drove her away. I say that because none of his old friends come around anymore either, like they did in the beginning. He is very rude and he makes people angry. The friends that he has now aren't really friends. They like him because he drinks with them. His behavior is childish and foolish. He talks about how he's going to do something with cars, fix them up and sell them but how can he with his handicap? I tell him that he ought to get some training in computers through a special program for handicapped people. He absolutely will not listen to anyone, especially to me. We argue all the time, and he does nothing but sit around and hang out with those hoods. I blame my separation partly on the fact that there is so much arguing. It's true that we had our problems but when my husband left a year ago, he said that no one could live in a nut house like this. He's living with his sister because she lives close to the shipyard where he works as a longshoreman. Once in a while he stops by to give me some money but he doesn't have much to do with his son. If the accident hadn't have happened and my son were living on his own, I think my husband would still be here. My son says he misses his father. After he left, he got real depressed. He said he wanted to kill himself. I think he wanted me to feel sorry for him even though he has no understanding about the way that I feel. He can't seem to understand or care about how anyone else feels but him. He is very self-centered. He wasn't that way before the accident.

My husband and I grew up in the same neighborhood in the city and let me tell you if any kid in that neighborhood acted like this, accident or no accident, he would have been out, just like that. Families didn't put up with it. All my brothers and sisters left home by the time they were 18. I had a brother and sister who got into trouble when they were 16 or around there. Out they went. They lived with friends. My mother didn't talk to my sister until the day she died. I don't see my family much but I know they would tell me to throw my son out and let him fend for himself. I guess I'm just soft-hearted. After all, he is sick. His memory is so bad that he'd probably get lost somewhere if he left the city. I had an uncle who had diabetes and his family didn't help him and he just gave up and died. Some people say that religion helps people through bad times like this. It didn't help my uncle and it's never helped me. I know that I'm the only person who cares what happens to my son. No one can help us. I'm just waiting for the worst to happen.

DISCUSSION QUESTIONS ON THE PERSONAL STATEMENT "...I'M JUST WAITING FOR THE WORST TO HAPPEN"

1. What kinds of stressors are created for the family when a person does not "learn" from an accident which has resulted in a head injury?

2. Should parents be "responsible" if their child does not wear a helmet?

3. How can a positive peer group be developed if a person's behavior isolates them?

4. How can threats of suicide be responded to constructively?

5. What helpful response could be made to this parent?

(SET 8)

RAIN OR SHINE

Perspective: One way to gain a perspective on the family challenged by a head injury is to explore how families in general and all families in particular function when life is ideal or not so ideal. Often, when families are in a state of crisis they lose contact with their pre-trauma reality and tend to believe that, prior to head trauma, their life was more functional, fulfilling and rewarding. Conversely, if the trauma did not occur, that their life would be more fulfilling, satisfying and rewarding.

Exploration:
1. List five qualities that define your family.
2. If you have experienced a head injury, were these qualities altered or changed?
3. If you were asked what are the abilities needed by a family to negotiate the perils of the head injury experience, what would they be?
4. Are the responses to a head injury different or similar to other traumas and losses?
5. Should divorce be considered as a reasonable alternative for persons married to a person with severe brain injury?
6. Should divorce be considered as a reasonable alternative for persons married to a person who has Alzheimer's Disease, AIDS, or a spinal cord injury?
7. Is the stress experienced by a family challenged by a head injury different that the stress related to other illnesses or disabilities? If so, in what ways?
8. Identify and discuss other familial factors that can intensify the stress associated with head injury.
9. Assuming that self-help and informational programs were available and accessible to families challenged by head injury, do you believe that all families would benefit from these resources?
10. Some families cope with the head injury experience by wanting, needing and perusing all relevant information. Other families see information as distressing and overwhelming. Do you feel that information is always helpful to families? If so, why? If not helpful, address.
11. If you were or are brain injured, what are or would be the sick role expectation your family have/would have for you?
12. Should people who are severely brain injured have their sexual needs and issues addressed by family members, as well as professionals?
13. How would your family respond if you were hypersexual and at risk to contract AIDS?

14. How would your family respond if you were married to a person with a severe head injury and you told them you were using alcohol to cope?

SET 9

I AM IN LOVE WITH A STRANGER

Perspective: Most relationships are based upon common goals, mutual respect, interpersonal concerns and emotional security. For those and a variety of other reasons, people choose to be with each other and enter a long-term relationship. Unfortunately, illness in general and head injury in particular can introduce elements into a relationship that are stressful, challenging and sometimes over-whelming. Some relationships can negotiate their challenges while others struggle and are eroded away.

Exploration:
1. Think of a couple you believe has an ideal relationship. How would this change if one of them experiences a head injury? Which one do you think could cope the best as a caregiver? As a patient?
2. If you know a couple who has successfully experienced a major trauma, discuss what enabled them to survive.

REFERENCES

Duvall, E. M. (1971). *Family development*. Philadelphia: J.B. Lippincott Co.

Jaffe, D. T. (1978). The role of family therapy in creating physical illness. *Hospital and Community Psychiatry, 29* (3), 169-174.

Keydel, C. F. (1991). *An exploration of perception and coping behavior in family members living with a closed head injured relative*. Unpublished doctoral dissertation, University of Maryland, College of Education, College Park.

Power, P. W., & Dell Orto, A. E. (1980). *Role of the family in the rehabilitation of the physically disabled*. Austin, TX: Pro-Ed.

Power, P. W., Dell Orto, A. E., & Gibbons, M. (1988). *Family intervention throughout chronic illness and disability*. New York: Springer Publishing Co.

Rakel, R. (1977). *Principles of family medicine*. Philadelphia: W.B. Saunders Co.

Rolland, J. S. (1988). A conceptual model of chronic and life- threatening illness and its impact on families. In C. Chilman, F. Cox, & E. Nunnally (Eds.), *Chronic illness and disability*. Newbury Park, CA: Sage Publications.

Warrington, J. (1981). *The Humpty Dumpty syndrome*. Light and Life Press. Available from the National Head Injury Foundation, Washington, D.C.

Zeigler, E. A. (1987, Jan/Feb/March). Spouses of persons who are brain injured. Journal of Rehabilitation, pp. 50-53.

5

FAMILY ASSESSMENT

5

FAMILY ASSESSMENT

The family is assuming a greater role in the treatment, adjustment, and rehabilitation of people with a head injury. Increased attention is being given to families in order to assist family members to learn how to adapt to and manage the disability within the family system (Brooks, Campsie, Symington, Beattie, & McKinlay, 1987; DeJong, Batavia, Williams, 1990; Durgin, 1989; Jacobs, 1984; Livingston & Brooks, 1988; McKinlay & Hickox, 1988; Quine, Pierce, & Lyle, 1988; Romano, 1974; Sachs, 1985; Schwentor & Brown, 1989).

For those available families who are involved in the life care management of a family member with a head-injury, a family assessment is often a key ingredient for developing an effective intervention and management plan. Also, family assessment should be an ongoing process because of the episodic nature of the effects of a head injury which may result in shifting family roles, and the sudden emergence of crisis situations. Therefore, it is important to understand the extent to which the family can support and follow through with specific management interventions in the home (Schwentor & Brown, 1989). A family assessment can also identify current functioning, the family member's expectations for recovery, and importantly, their needs for services. In other words, an assessment with the family is an information-obtaining approach that establishes the foundation for appropriate intervention (Kreutzer, Leininger, Doherty, & Waaland, 1987; Kreutzer, Camplair, & Waaland, 1988).

There are many ways to conduct a family assessment. Some of these include standardized and quantifiable methods such as a self-report, which employs questionnaires that ask for an individual's perception of the family's functioning (Bishop & Miller, 1988). Another approach is observation which occurs when the family is observed in the home carrying out assigned tasks that are designed specifically for the family. Still another family assessment method is interviewing the family in the home setting. An assessment conducted in the home enables the interviewer to evaluate areas such as individual dynamics, family interaction, living arrangements, environment, and resources. With everyone assembled in the home, communication can be encouraged among family members, and the nature of problems arising from the head injury can be discussed openly. On their own "turf," family members are usually more open to the interviewer, more prone to discuss their disability related problems, and more ready to share information. If possible, all family members who are living in the home, or who have almost immediate availability to the family home, should be included when the interview is being conducted. At the beginning of any family assessment, the interviewer may be unaware of those persons who have a decided influence on the management of the person with a head injury. Someone who is missing from the assessment interview could be that person who has a dominating influence on the person with a head injury or the family process and who could influence treatment and rehabilitation outcomes.

While doing a family assessment, it is helpful for the interviewer to follow structured guidelines. In an article focusing on the assessment of families with a brain-injured member, Schwentor and Brown (1989) stress the need for "multiple methods, tools and sources of information." (p.13).

AN ASSESSMENT APPROACH

In order to be effective and relevant while working with the family coping with a head injury, the health and human care professional should understand the dynamics that are unique to each family. The following general assessment approach explores this information, and focuses on the unique characteristics of the family. It can identify those areas of family life that may be negatively influencing the patient's adjustment, and, in turn, indicate those factors in the family constellation that could promote the adaptation of family members.

The following information represents suggested family assessment guidelines which can serve as an outline when taking a family history.

I.   Family Demographic Information and Other Considerations
      A. Age and gender of family members
      B. Occupation of spouses and family
      C. Educational background of parents and siblings
      D. Ethnicity
      E. Religion
      F. How many family members contribute to the family income?
      G. How long has the family lived in its present location?
      H. Are relatives living nearby and available in time of crisis?
      I. Who pays the bills in the family?

    J.   Does the family have adequate medical insurance coverage?

    K. What are the family plans for the future concerning:
1. education
2. vacation
3. retirement

    L.   What are the current and future major expenses of the family?

    M. Any prior experience with head injury?

    N.   What is the primary role of the person with a head injury in the family group? For example, is this person left out from family planning?

    O. Are there other serious family problems (e.g., alcoholism or drug abuse, mental illness or other stressors)? How is it connected with the patient's medical or rehabilitation problems?

    P.   Who is working? What are work hours? How much work related stress exists?

II.   **Communication Patterns in the Family**

    A. Is there open hostility among family members?

    B. Do the family members appear to provide emotional support for each other? How is this support given?

    C. What activities do family members share together?

    D. Who dominates the family discussions? Who most frequently contradicts the dominant influence?

    E. Do all family members express their opinions readily or is someone the spokesperson for the family?

    F. Do individual schedules permit much time together at home as a family?

    G. What are the communication of feelings toward the person coping with head injury?

    H. How would one describe the sibling relationship?

    I.   Are there any current areas of family satisfaction?

    J.   Is there any communication with extended family

III.   **Division of Labor in the Family**

    A. What was the role of parents and children in the family before head injury: what is to be done, who is to do it, and who takes leadership in deciding on allocation of tasks

    B. What kinds of things are people expected to do around the house?

    C. Which family members work together?

    D. As a result of the head injury, have family roles remained flexible or rigid? What role shifts have occurred?

    E. Who is responsible for transportation?

IV. **Extent of Family Members' Outside Socialization and Access to Social and Cultural Experiences**
   A. Quantity
   B. Quality

V. **Health or Illness**
   A. Do family members have regular clinic or doctor appointments?
   B. Any previous serious illness/disabilities in the family? If so, what are the family members' feelings about their experiences with doctors and hospitals?
   C. What are the general attitudes toward pain, loss, disability, treatment plans, or a specific illness? For example, do family members believe that the particular illness is amenable to treatment, or that treatment will lead to better health?

VI. **Characteristics of the Head Injury**
   A. What are the physical and emotional consequences of head injury?
   B. What was the age of the person when the head injury occurred?
   C. How is the person limited emotionally, physically, intellectually and vocationally?
   D. What was the cause of the head injury? Situation, circumstances, and responsibility.
   E. What do the family members and the patient understand about the nature and implications of head injury?
   F. What are the attitudes of significant others toward head injury?
   G. What are the family members' perception of the future limiting aspects of the patient as a result of head injury?

VII. **Impact of Head Injury on the Family**
   A. Impact on the regular performance of duties within the home?
   B. Impact on the activities of family members outside of the home?
   C. Do the family members identify any continued adjustment problems resulting from the head injury?
   D. Are community agencies used? Do they seem to be adequate?
   E. What are expectations of family members for each other?
      1. Toward household duties
      2. Maintaining social contacts
      3. Vocational goals
   F. How have the family members accepted the financial restrictions, if any, imposed by the head injury?
   G. What is the perception of family members about their resources in dealing with the head injury?

    H. How does each family member describe how they are dealing with the presence of head injury in the family?

    I. How have family members in previous family generations handled illness and disability situations?

    J. Who do family members believe is the best person to care for the person with a head injury?

    K. Has there been a realignment of family goals?

    L. Has there been a change in the social needs of family members?

    M. Do family members' refer to past areas of satisfaction, including previous successful experiences with crises.

    N. Is there a great deal of guilt, shame, and feelings of frustration among family members?

VIII. **Appraisal of the residual health of the family relationships**
    A. What areas of the marital and parental interaction and shared functioning are least damaged?
    B. What areas are most damaged?

IX. **Appraisal of the damage of the relationships resulting from the adjustment to head injury**
    A. Does head injury threaten to engulf all major aspects of the marital and parental interactions, or are its effects relatively circumscribed?
    B. Are there clear signs of a push toward isolation, disintegration, or regression in the family relationships?

CONCLUSION

In response to many of these assessment areas, family members may have difficulty in being precise in their answers. Yet the interviewer should ask the family members to elaborate on their responses, at the same time being sensitive to the feelings of family members. The family may be resistant to any intervention efforts, and support and reassurance should be given to help comfort and reinforce the family for their own caregiving efforts. Moreover, special consideration should be given to the presence of other stressors that are not directly related to the head injury situation (other family health problems, unemployment). It is also important to consider that interviews with extended family members may provide useful intergenerational information in identifying both strengths and problems in the family (Schwentor & Brown, 1989). A major contribution in the area of interviewing is the current research on the Head Injury Family Interview (Hi-Fi) which is being developed by the Research and Training Center on Head Trauma and Stroke at the New York University Medical Center (Kay, Cavallo, & Ezrachi,1993).

There are many challenges in implementing a viable and reasonable treatment-rehabilitation plan for families and persons who are living with the impact of head injury. A primary step in this process is an assessment approach that is responsive to the many influences that impact the head injured family member, the total family system, and their mutual needs.

The following personal statement, "We're Tough," explores the impact of a severe head injury on familial roles, the ongoing stress related to coping and surviving, as well as the power of a religious-cultural perspective.

Personal Statement

... WE'RE TOUGH
(A Wife's Perspective)

I am a 45-year-old woman whose husband of 24 years suffered a traumatic brain injury three years ago. At the time of his injury, we lived in a large house in the suburb of a midwestern city surrounded by other families of the orthodox Jewish faith. I was preparing for the empty nest and had gone to college to get a degree in interior decoration. Our older daughter was in her senior year in college and our younger daughter in her senior year in high school. I was going to have a lot of time on my hands with the girls gone and I was looking forward to having a career and to spending more time with my husband. He was an executive in an accounting firm and very busy with work and with his involvement in our temple. Everyone admired and respected him but he had very little time to spend at home. He had promised to give up some of his religious activities and spend more time with me. Little did I know that soon he would be spending all his time with me and it wouldn't be happy time!

Our lives changed drastically one night three years ago. It was a winter night and slippery out. I tried to convince my husband to cancel his meeting that night; he insisted on going but promised to come home early. The next thing I knew I was rushing to our local hospital emergency ward where I was told that he had been in a bad collision and had suffered a severe head injury and probably wouldn't live. For days he hovered between life and death. The whole Jewish community prayed for him. He was in a coma for three weeks but he lived. When he finally woke up, it was like a miracle, but we weren't prepared for the way that he was. He tried to hit the nurses and said things to people that he never would have said before the accident. He was a stranger. My daughters couldn't take it. They didn't want to go to the hospital. After the acute phase, he was in the rehabilitation hospital for six months and finally he came home. I think I neglected my daughters during that time. I feel bad about that. All I could think about was my husband and they never got the attention that children should get when they're in their senior year. They don't say anything about it but I think they resent the fact that I wasn't excited about their activities. I couldn't even get involved in my younger daughter's trip to Israel that summer. But what about me? One day I have a husband who is the strength of the family, who makes everyone proud and the next, I have this person who scares everyone with his temper and who thinks everything is fine when it's a sorry mess.

Life is getting better. The two of us get along. Sometimes I even like the fact that my husband is around all the time. He can be good company. But he can also be very difficult, almost impossible at times. He has a lot of anger and frustration but he won't face that yet; he still has trouble controlling his temper; he says whatever he is thinking and frequently insults people. His daughters do not like to stay with him alone because he tries to do things that are dangerous for him to do like walking outside without his cane and when they try to talk him out of it, he gets furious, says insulting things to them and does whatever he pleases. He can't face reality yet. He wants to go back to work but he can't remember from one minute to the next. He is still very intelligent but in the middle of what you think is a very reasonable comment, he'll say something foolish, but he doesn't realize it. He thinks that he is making good sense. You can't tell him anything in a critical way; he becomes a "crazy man."

We had to move to a one story house, out of our old neighborhood. That was also very hard on the girls. Fortunately, my husband's business had excellent health insurance so we didn't have to go into debt. They also had a good disability plan and we can just live on it but things are very tight. Everyone says I should get someone to stay with my husband so I can go out, but do you have any idea what that costs? Besides, I wouldn't trust most people to know how to handle him, especially when he's difficult. The girls think that I should get him to go to a therapist. They think that he could be helped to control his temper and to remember better. Maybe I will one of these days. Health insurance would help pay for that. I recently joined a support group. It feels like I am associating with a whole new social group, people who are down and out, so to speak. I joined because I hoped that it would be a way to find out about community resources for the head injured. There doesn't seem to be much out there. Some people in the support group trade respite care with each other but I don't think my husband would like spending time with a stranger. They wouldn't have anything in common. I'm particularly worried about the future when I get too old to take care of him. Of course my daughters will always be available but they'll have their own families and their father would be an extra burden for them. I would never put him in a home unless I absolutely had to.

I guess we'll be a good old twosome until the day we die. Once in a great while, I do things with my friends and I have my needlework. I'm not unhappy. I'm a survivor. My ancestors were all tough, let me tell you. Life is hard. I'm a survivor.

DISCUSSION QUESTIONS ON THE PERSONAL STATEMENT "WE'RE TOUGH"

1. Reflecting on the assessment approach discussed in this chapter, what important issues emerge in this personal statement?

2. How does religion impact coping with a head injury?

3. What are the unique stressors related to the onset of a parental head injury when a couple has reached the end of the child rearing stage?

4. What did the wife mean by the statement, "He was a stranger."? How does this reality challenge the resources of the non-injured spouse?

5. Discuss the "advantages" and disadvantages of having a person with a head injury around all of the time?

6. How can a family protect a person with a head injury while trying to have them live as independently as possible?

7. How would this family cope if they did not have excellent health insurance?

8. What are the factors to be considered when developing a long-range plan that meets the needs of the person who has a head injury as well as the needs of the primary caregiver?

9. How can traditions and cultural expectations be an asset or a liability?

(SET 10)

GOOD FEELINGS, BAD FEELINGS

Perspective: To present awareness that families have different attitudes and feelings to each other individually and or collectively. This is an important point to consider when addressing the needs of the person with a head injury as well as the family. For example, all persons with a head injury do not love their spouse, children, and or family. Similarly, not all families love, care about, or want to respond to the needs of a person with a head injury. The following questions will facilitate discussion of this point and identify many areas that are critical in the assessment process.

Exploration:
1. How should a family respond to their mother who abandoned them 20 years ago and now is seeking a reconciliation since she was in a car accident and had severe head injury.
2. What would you advise a friend whose brain injured parent sexually abused him/her as a child and now wants to move in so he/she can be with the grandchildren.
3. What should a wife do to meet the needs of her brain injured sister who paid her tuition so she could go to medical school. An additional factor is her husband dislikes his sister-in-law since her brain injury and said he would leave if his wife wants to get involved.

4. What should a child do when his/her mother remarries and after one year her new husband has severe head injury? This is complicated by the fact that mother left her first husband because she could not deal with his head injury, consequently, the children took care of their father until he committed suicide.

5. Identify and discuss the community resources available in your area that could meet the needs of your family if you experienced a severe head injury.

6. If you experienced a head injury today, how would you accept and cope with the losses?

7. Would family responses to your head injury be different today than it would have been 10 years ago? Why?

8. What kind of information related to head injury would be helpful to you and your family?

9. What kind of information would not be helpful?

10. How would your family respond if you were unable to "adjust" to your head injury and you became a source of conflict in the family?

11. In what way does ethnic background impact the families response to loss or head injury?

12. What are the problems and needs of a family that must deal with other stressors such as alcoholism while living with a family member who is head injured?

13. What activities can a post-injury family engage in to promote a quality of life?

14. What would a home visit by a health care worker reveal about your family?

15. What are your family's fondest memories?

16. How would a head injury to a family member alter your family's goals?

17. What emotions would your family have a difficult time sharing?

18. What family values would you want to be part of your future?

19. Have these or would these values assist you in coping with the demands and losses associated with a head injury?

20. Who in your family could cope with a major loss with the best attitude? Why?

REFERENCES

Bishop, D. S., & Miller, I. W. (1988). Traumatic brain injury: Empirical family assessment techniques. *Journal of Head Trauma Rehabilitation, 3, 4,* 16-30.

Brooks, N., Campsie, L., Symington, C., Beattie, A., & McKinlay, W. (1987). The effects of severe brain injury on patient and relative within seven years of injury. *Journal of Head Trauma Rehabilitation, 2(3),* 1-13.

DeJong, G., Batavia, A. I., & Williams, J. M. (1990). Who is responsible for the lifelong well being of a person with a head injury? *Journal of Head Trauma Rehabilitation, 5(1),* 9-22.

Durgin, C. J. (1989, May-June). Techniques for families to increase their involvement in the rehabilitation process. *Cognitive Rehabilitation* , pp. 22-25.

Jacobs, H. E. (1984). *The family as a therapeutic agent: Long term rehabilitation for traumatic head injury patients.* Final report of the Mary Switzer Research Fellowship, 1983-1984. National Institute of Handicapped Research.

Kay, T., Cavallo, M. M., & Ezrachi, O. (1993). *Administration manual, N.Y.U. head injury family interview (Version 2.0).* New York: N.Y.U. Medical Center, Research and Training Center on Head Trauma and Stroke.

Kreutzer, J., Leininger, B., Doherty, K., & Waaland, P. (1987). *General health and history questionnaire.* Richmond: Medical College of Virginia, Rehabilitation Research and Training Center on Severe Traumatic Brain Injury.

Kreutzer, J., Camplair, P., & Waaland, P. (1988). *Family needs questionnaire.* Richmond: Medical College of Virginia, Rehabilitation Research and Training Center on Severe Traumatic Brain Injury.

Livingston, M. G., & Brooks, D. N. (1988). The burden on families of the brain injured: A review. *Journal of Head Trauma Rehabilitation, 3(4),* 6-15.

McKinlay, W., & Hickox, A. (1988). How can families help in the rehabilitation of the head injured? *Journal of Head Trauma Rehabilitation, 3(4),* 64-72.

Quine, S., Pierce, J. P., & Lyle, D. M. (1988). Relatives as lay- therapists for the severely head-injured. *Brain Injury, 2,* 139-149.

Romano, M. D. (1974). Family response to traumatic head injury. *Scandinavian Journal of Rehabilitation Medicine, 6,* 1-5.

Sachs, P. R. (1985). Beyond support: Traumatic head injury as a growth experience for families. *Rehabilitation Nursing, 10(1),* 21-23.

Schwentor, D., & Brown, P. (1989, May/June). Assessment of families with a traumatically brain-injured relative. *Cognitive Rehabilitation,* pp. 8-14.

6

HEAD INJURY AND FAMILY INTERVENTION

6

HEAD INJURY AND FAMILY INTERVENTION

Many specific interventions for the person with a head injury have been recently identified (Hart & Jacobs, 1993; Marmé & Skord, 1993; Medlar, 1993). This awareness supports the families play a significant role in both the present and future life of the person with head injury. Many families find themselves providing perpetual care and treatment to a "transformed" family member. For family members the behavioral, emotional, and cognitive problems are usually the most difficult to manage, and the hidden financial, physical, and emotional costs associated with caring for a head injured survivor often impairs or even destroys the family unit (Jacobs, 1984). Helping a family adjust to the impact of a head injury requires an appropriate course of action, and through this intervention caregivers can be helped to function more effectively and efficiently in their demanding and changing roles.

The struggle by family members to achieve adaptive roles involves an ongoing process of dealing with the many problems that result from living with a person with head injury. These problems include the possible social isolation of family members, the constant demand to carry out the prescribed treatment regimen, managing the family member's own grief, dealing with unpredictable behavior, and assuming the burden of caregiving responsibilities (Zeigler, 1989). Also, the continued inclination to become overinvolved with the person with head injury, and the ever-present reality that the person with head injury might draw attention away from other marital and family needs should be considered.

The following chapters, Chapters 6, 7, and 8, explore different intervention strategies. All three chapters focus on the alleviation of problems, as well as optimizing opportunities generated by living with a person with a head injury. The overall goal is to support the family, as well as to help family members minimize their own disability-related problems. Chapter 6 identifies theoretical assumptions for intervention, particular intervention goals for families attempting to adjust to the head injury trauma, and then specific tasks to accomplish these goals. Yet within these intervention considerations that apply to most families as they live with the person who is gradually meeting treatment and rehabilitation objectives, there are specific situations which necessitate a particular helping approach. These situations, which are generated when living the head injury experience, are unexpected family crises and stress of coping with the reality of permanent loss. Both of these realities call for special skills when developing a helping approach, and these are discussed in Chapters 7 and 8. Because crisis and loss and grief present complex situations for the helping professional and family members, these two chapters build on the material presented in Chapter 6 and then give the reader guidelines for assisting families in these different situations.

THEORETICAL ASSUMPTIONS

For an intervention approach to be effective, there are certain assumptions critical to an intervention with families of persons with a head injury.

1. **An intervention effort directed toward the person and family is a joint venture shared by the health care and rehabilitation professional and the family members.** If the person, family members, and professional worker share their energy and resources, it will facilitate the attainment of common goals. It is important to emphasize that the family is an integral part of the helping process, and most individuals cannot be treated in isolation even if they are severely limited by a head injury. If they become a partner in intervention, stabilization, and rehabilitation efforts, the family members generally develop more willingness to work with each other. This is particularly true when family members choose between competing goals and values as they attempt to cope with the reality of head injury. The degree of consensus that develops among family members regarding the ranking of family goals can be a crucial factor in the family's ability to deal successfully with adjustment demands. What often fosters this consensus is the mutuality that has already been established between the health care worker and the family.

2. **There will be predictable points of family stress when coping with head injury.** Each of these periods must be examined individually, because each can bring unique problems. For example, discharge planning can surface many unre-

solved issues regarding family roles during the rehabilitation process. Also, additional problems can be created when the person with a head injury is at home because caring responsibilities may force family members to assume different functions in the home.

3. **The basic instinct of people under stress is to hold to previously proved patterns of action, whether they are effective or not.** A family reactive pattern will usually not vary too much from the way that family members have responded in the past. Health care professionals should make an effort during family assessment to understand these past adjustment styles and be aware of how they influence the present.

4. **Rehabilitation is generally a process of teaching persons to live with their disability in their own environment.** The key to coping with one's disability is to receive enough satisfactions and rewards to make life worthwhile (Treischmann, 1974). When reinforcements for the person are withdrawn from the family environment, he or she may feel isolated and become reluctant to respond to treatment efforts, or may become more manipulative in attempts to gain attention. The complexity of head injury is that the family must accept the loss of the preinjury person and accept the new person in the family. For some family systems this is a manageable task; for others it is an illusive dream or an unending nightmare.

5. **Intervention programs that aim to increase caregiver's knowledge and/or perceived social support can consist of presentations, discussion groups, and support groups.** A multi-dimensional approach that emphasizes the acquisition of caregiver skills through periodic interaction with those who have experience in dealing with head injury within the family can assist family members to manage the different problems resulting from the disability. Further, those caregivers who have been socialized to be more passive and accepting of things as they are, may benefit from a support group that provides role models as well as skills related to living in spite of stress, loss, and trauma. (Appendices A and B)

Emerging from these assumptions are specific goals for family intervention. Family adaptation to head injury is ongoing and will stimulate varied family reactions and different adjustment demands. During the unfolding process of family adjustment, there are certain adaptive goals which are ever-present and which provoke definite tasks for goal achievement by family members. They are:

PROVIDING THE FAMILY WITH A SENSE OF COMPETENCE

The occurrence of a head injury will increase anxiety for family members as well as reinforce feelings of sadness, guilt, confusion, isolation, anger, and helplessness. An intervention approach should aid family members to alleviate these feelings and to assist them to regain or develop control of their lives, individually and collectively. The development of such competence usually represents the creation of new, positive family influences on the individual with a head injury.

The tasks to achieve these competencies include:

a. Learning about the effects of a head injury and the implications for physical, emotional, and intellectual functioning.
b. Learning how to deal with varied management problems accruing from the head injury.
c. Learning different coping strategies that assist family members to handle more effectively daily living concerns.
d. Learning how to interact effectively with health professionals and/or members of the rehabilitation team.
e. Learning problem solving skills.
f. Learning, when necessary, how to make necessary shifts in role responsibilities.

ASSISTING THE FAMILY TO NORMALIZE RELATIONS WITH EACH OTHER AND, AS MUCH AS POSSIBLE, WITH THE FAMILY MEMBER EXPERIENCING A HEAD INJURY

Normalization is an effort to provide appropriate patterns of expectations from family members for continued activities and maintenance of customary role responsibilities. Normalization does not eliminate the possibility, however, that many families will have to become re-oriented to the realities of the head injury. For family members the problem is usually not head injury as an abstract concept, but how to cope with it in every critical aspect of their lives.

The tasks that assist family members to achieve normalization include:

a. Give responsibility, when appropriate, to the person for appropriate home duties and a voice in family matters.
b. Understand their own grief reaction, and that such feelings as fear of the future, anger, frustration and disappointment are to be expected among family members.
c. Understand their own perception of what the head injury means to family life, and to discuss this perception, when appropriate, with other family members.

   d.   Balance the needs of the person with a head injury with the needs of other family members.

   e.   Learn to take care of themselves, their significant others, and their marriage.

DEVELOPING A RENEWED AWARENESS BY FAMILY MEMBERS OF THEIR OWN RESOURCES AND STRENGTHS

In their attempts to manage the effects of the head injury on family life, family members often overlook their own assets and strengths in dealing with recurrent problems. The stress induced from living with a person with a head injury frequently stimulates a continued family state of anxiety, which, in turn, clouds the identification of those capabilities which can lead to this awareness.

Tasks that can assist family members to attain this goal are:

   a.   An understanding of how past family crises were handled, and a recognition of transgenerational coping strategies.

   b.   Utilize community resources, especially participation in support groups which can provide feedback to family members on their own capabilities.

   c.   Enhance their own expectations for each other regarding family tasks and management responsibilities for head injury.

   d.   Communicate with each other about their own needs and their own concerns in living with head injury.

CREATING A CONSISTENT, SUPPORTIVE, EMOTIONAL EXPERIENCE FOR THE FAMILY IN WHICH THEIR MUTUAL NEEDS AND FEELINGS ARE RECOGNIZED AND ACKNOWLEDGED

Frequently the multidimensionality of losses experienced by the person with a head injury (e.g., those caused by physical restrictions or loss of job due to head injury) are overlooked by other family members. The person with a head injury may be hesitant to talk about personal losses because one perceives that other family members will not understand, or will be overwhelmed. Instead, these feelings are suppressed or the person reacts to this family unresponsiveness by exaggerated dependency or continual irritation with others. To create this supportive experience for the family the following tasks can be considered:

   a.   Learn how to talk with each other, in the family, about their own concerns and needs, and provide an atmosphere for this discussion when these feelings, concerns, and needs will not be negatively evaluated.

   b.   Foster the awareness of mutual respect and recognition of each family member's self-worth.

The focus for all of these identified tasks is on the emerging needs of the family. If the family is to be an important resource in the treatment and/or rehabilitation of the head injured family member, then family members will have to acquire certain skills. Each task implies the utilization of an accompanying skill, and apart from the imparting of necessary information to family members about head injury, much of the intervention efforts will deal with assisting family members to acquire these skills. What skills families need will depend on what has been learned from the family assessment. Also, how emotional problems relevant to the family's living with the effects of the head injury are resolved depends on the nature of the problem and its relationship to the trauma. Head injury alters the family structure, and, consequently, communication patterns can change.

Intervention can be conducted by rehabilitation and health care professionals or by non-professionals-peers and family. Intervention often begins when a member of the patient's rehabilitation team contacts a professional for possible family assistance. Frequently the rehabilitation team encourages family members to seek short-term assistance in order to deal with both expected and unexpected problems. The family visits may take place either in an office or home setting, and if initiated soon after the onset of head injury, should take place as often as possible in order to alleviate family concerns. Intervention by non-professionals usually takes place in a support group setting, and the rehabilitation team may recommend such an opportunity as the individual is undergoing in-patient treatment and family concerns are emerging. Usually family members do not seek a support group until they are confronted with serious family problems and they realize that input from others and the ventilation of their feelings will assist in their own adjustment efforts.

With this focus on the family's acquisition of adaptive skills, or tasks, there are three approaches that can be beneficial for helping families both to learn and to implement the skills. These three approaches are counseling, education, and support. Again, whether the approach is primarily counseling, education, or support will depend on what is learned about family needs during the assessment process.

COUNSELING

This intervention is usually oriented to current family functioning, and involves such approaches as providing family members with the opportunity to share their feelings with each other, learning important information about the head injury process, asking for clarification of issues and encouraging questions that lead to an understanding of how family members perceive the injury affecting family life and their own expectations. One of the initial goals of counseling, before formal education approaches or formal supports are suggested, is to assist the family members to have trust in the health or human care provider, as well as to assist the family members to understand their own perception of their ability and willingness to provide care for the person with the head injury and to take care of themselves during the treatment and/or rehabilitation process. Because of the importance for the achievement of these goals, the provider should begin a counseling intervention with the family as soon as it is possible after the onset of the head injury. While the individual is undergoing critical care management in the hospital, family members usually need to have questions answered, be reassured, and be told that someone is available to act as a resource for their own emerging problems. In counseling family members attempts are made to maintain a listening, non-evaluative posture which encourages the expression of feelings and questions by the family. The service provider needs to develop trust with the family, and often this can be generated by the professional's acceptance of family feelings and showing a genuine interest to assist family members. Counseling also includes helping families to recognize their own strengths and specific problem areas, sharing information about the head injury and varied management issues, and perhaps preparing the family for possible events related to the head injury that eventually may be of concern to the family.

When considering such process counseling issues as listening, encouraging the expression of questions and emotions, and identifying central problem areas, then counseling continues during the entire span of intervention. The interventions of support and education imply that the process of counseling is still an on-going reality with the family members.

EDUCATION

As a vitally important intervention approach, education can take a number of forms. For example, many rehabilitation treatment centers and other related agencies have formal education programs for family members. During these programs information about head injury is imparted, family questions are answered, and management techniques are suggested that can deal with such problems as poor attention span, inappropriate social skills, low frustration tolerance, and disorientation and organizational problems. Different community resources are also identified. Many families can benefit from these programs, since family members can learn problem solving skills from personnel who usually are extremely knowledgeable about the implications of head injury for family life. The role of the service provider is helping the family to utilize formal and informal education opportunities. With the knowledge of what education programs are available, the provider can indicate the advantages to family members from their involvement in these activities. (See Appendix E.)

Frequently, however, the health care provider must assume the role of educator since the family may not have the immediate opportunity to take part in any formal program, or, information must be imparted that responds to current problems. This information can include a wide scope of topics, such as the availability of community resources, the nature of head injury and the implications of cognitive, emotional, and behavioral deficits on patient and family functioning, the teaching of effective coping skills, insights into how family expectations may have to change, and ways that family members can take care of themselves and their marriage. Financial and legal information may also be included, as well as sharing with the family how issues of blame and guilt can be managed. Education can further include the identification to the family how previous family generations have handled family crises, and what coping resources can be utilized during the present crisis. (See Appendix A, B, and C)

The teaching of coping skills is a particularly valuable education contribution that health and human care providers can make to the family's own adjustment efforts. Coping itself comprises efforts to manage stressful demands, regardless of outcome. There are many threats and challenges to family life as the result of the head injury trauma, and families need to evaluate the range of their own coping resources and alternatives. One particular coping strategy during the family's adjustment to head injury is reframing, namely, attempting to see the patient's behavior in a different light. A family member, through reframing, gives another meaning to the situation. This meaning can be attained by positive comparisons by recognizing even some of the patient's negative behaviors as signs of patient progress, or by becoming convinced that eventually the burdens accruing from patient management and care will diminish. Reframing involves, therefore, changing one's attitude, focusing on caregiving strengths, and even creating one's own system of affective rewards. Other coping approaches may include the reliance for strength on one's religious faith, sharing concerns with others, seeking as much information as possible about the injury and its implications for the future, patient functioning, and undertaking rational problem solving. This problem solving entails talking out the problem, looking at choices, when these are available, and then developing a plan of action to confront and minimize the problem.

Another aspect of educational intervention is teaching family members how to deal and work with health care and rehabilitation professionals. Because of their own anxiety and unfamiliarity with all the issues of head injury, family members may tend to be reluctant to ask questions, or to be more assertive during the interactions with the rehabilitation team. Families can be taught to record carefully the different treatment plans that will be undertaken with the injured family member, to ask health professionals to repeat unclear statements, and to be assertive in seeking information about certain problems that arise as treatment continues. If the family is to negotiate successfully the problems of living with someone with head injury, then questions arising from adjustment and treatment concerns must be asked. Assertiveness and self-advocacy by family members can stimulate the communication, as well as the mutual awareness process. A suggested educational program that explores these issues is presented in Appendix E.

SUPPORT

There are many operational definitions of support, such as the expression of emotional support (esteem, affect, trust); the communication of appraisal support (affirmation, feedback); giving information (advice, suggestions); and providing instrumental support (money, labor, time) (House, 1981). All of these types of support apply to families experiencing the trauma of head injury, and such support can be provided either by an individual worker or by family support groups. The latter resource frequently addresses the issues faced by family members with a desire to speak with someone dealing with their own unique collection of problems. Barker (1988) describes the need for involvement with other spouses:

> The only way you can cope with it is to talk with someone who understands, has experienced the same thing, and knows just what the situation is, so that all you have to do sometimes is just say a few words and the other person knows exactly what you're talking about without going into all the details. (In Zeigler, 1989, p.36)

In family head injury situations, families with good support systems appear to be more successful in overcoming traumatic situations and maintaining a family sense of competence. Keydel (1991), in studying families living with head injury, reported that it was the belief that support was available rather than the use of support that was contributing to the alleviation of family stress. Another influence on the perception of social support is the family's belief about the acceptability of asking for support from others. Getting help from others may be perceived in some families as a testimony to the strength and closeness of the family and friendship network; or, the effects of the head injury on the family may be so traumatizing that family members, in their low feelings of self-esteem, may believe they are not entitled to support, may not ask for it, or may even refuse it when offered (Keydel, 1991).

The timing of providing support, especially in the forms of giving information or urging family members to become involved in family support groups, needs to be handled carefully. In the early stages of head injury many family members may still need the protective shield of denial, and would consequently find information and support groups quite negative. Family members need to feel comfortable when hearing about problems which might still exist many years down the road (Zeigler, 1989). Intervention approaches which emphasize support should then consider the needs of family members and when the communication of information, or hearing how others have dealt with problems, would be most appropriately received.

Whether support takes the form of feedback, reassurance, or advice, the communication of support is an active process that acknowledges the family's abilities and reinforces those aspects of the family's functioning that appear adaptive and beneficial to the treatment process. Support includes helping family members to search or understand how they are reacting to the trauma, encouraging the expression of family feelings, and helping family members to make active decisions in daily care (Sachs, 1991).

Conclusion

Whether intervention is primarily counseling, education, or support, it should enable families to attain and maintain a reasonable quality of life. At the same time as they perform their caregiving roles, the family acts as a resource for the potential rehabilitation, growth and development of the transformed family member. Intervention should be tailored to the individual needs of families and focus on aiding family members to bring their life back to normal as they respond to caregiving demands. Efforts to regain the balance in family life requires a sense of competency by family members, a consistent emotional experience for the family, and an awareness of their own strengths, limitations, and resources.

The following personal statement, "One More Burden," presents the challenges faced by a mother whose dreams were shattered. It reflects the complexity of loss, as well as an emerging optimism for the future based upon a unique perspective formulated in difficult circumstances.

Personal Statement

... ONE MORE BURDEN
(A Mother's Perspective)

I am a 51-year-old black woman who lives with my daughter in a small house in a quiet section of a Southern City. I worked as a kitchen helper for many years, but have been unemployed because of serious illnesses and disabilities. I suffer from asthma and a heart condition, and receive S.S.I. I walk with great difficulty and am not able to go up the stairs in my home. I also have two other daughters who live nearby. They both have children; one has completed the 11th grade, but is now unemployed and is receiving Aid to Families with Dependent Children. My other daughter has completed the ninth grade, is unemployed and is receiving also Aid to Families with Dependent Children. Both daughters with their children were living with me until the serious accident of my other daughter.

My daughter, 25 years old, was driving her car and was thrown into the windshield when she was hit from behind by a car that ran a stop light. She was not wearing her seatbelt at the time of the accident. She suffered a serious head injury and spent many, many months in the hospital. When they discharged her, she came to live with me, and my two daughters had to move out. Since she has been at home, she has been unemployed and has received medical certification that she is permanently disabled and unemployable. She tells me that she has a short-term memory impairment and she has these frequently- occurring seizures, which really scare me. All my family members are Baptists and we have strong religious beliefs, and God will get us through this. My daughter has tried to work for short periods of time, but has been unable to do so because of severe memory problems.

Before the accident, my daughter was a very good girl, had a good job, her own apartment, and was dating a man who eventually left her after the accident. She was involved in gospel singing at the church. Now my daughter helps me around the house, though it always seems dirty. My daughters come over quite frequently to see us, and I think they are resentful of my daughter because they had to move out when she left the hospital. But because of my sickness, I was not able to manage all of them under the same roof. I also have many friends, my church, and they are a support to me during this trial.

None of the family believe that my daughter was at fault for the accident, though they both wonder why she was not wearing her seatbelt on the day of the accident. Yet I believe that I told my daughter the morning of the accident that she should always wear her seatbelt, even if she was driving close to home. If she had done all of this, this accident might not have happened and she would not be limited as she is now. But I guess we all really believe that the accident had just happened and not for any reason. Yet all of us believe that our sister and daughter was such a good person before the accident. We were very impressed with her lifestyle–a nice apartment with fine furniture and plants everywhere. In our eyes, she was a successful person, and a very quiet person. Now after the accident we think she is thinner and even more energetic. Yet I don't say "energy" in the positive sense. She really has changed for the worse. Funny, but I think my daughter is still attractive, hopeful, caring and friendly, but my other daughters think she is more irritable and even a troublemaker. They think that, though she was not the youngest, she acts like she is the baby in the family. Yet my injured daughter does not share in these beliefs, as she feels that she has not changed that much, though she realizes that she is more dependent on all of us, and she has even said that she is less attractive now. After living with my daughter now for several months, I don't think she is going to change too much. We all hope that she gets much better, but I wonder about that.

The most stressful part of our family life now is living with the seizures. We just can't do anything about them, and I worry that they might be fatal and I also worry that I might have a heart attack because of the stress. "When I get upset, I get chest pains." When we are all here and she has a seizure, we pray together that she will come out of it. We panic, but we do roll her over from side to side to keep her from swallowing her tongue. Because of these seizures happening at unknown times, and I believe that I cannot manage the situation, my daughters come over very often just in case a seizure might happen. But you know, I get a "funny feelings" when a seizure might happen, and I had that feeling the day of the accident. I expect the seizures will get worse, and I don't know what I can do about it.

Deep down I think it is good for me to have my daughter at home. My friends seem to come in here all the time, as we have been living here for many, many years. My husband died many years ago. I believe that families should take care of each other. I am fine if my children are all right, so right now I am not so fine because of this head injury business. I took care of my mother when she was dying and I expect my children will take care of me just as I care for them. I can manage if we have this togetherness. All the doctors are necessary, but it is family that really counts. But this seizure business is getting the best of all of us, but we just group together and do the best we can. God will take care of us.

DISCUSSION QUESTIONS ON THE PERSONAL STATEMENT "ONE MORE BURDEN"

1. Whose "fault" was the accident?

2. Is it more difficult to let go of a "productive" pre-injured person?

3. What are the issues generated by wearing and not wearing a seatbelt?

4. Why are the seizures a source of stress?

5. What are the futuristic concerns in the situation?

6. How can a religious perspective be helpful in coping with a head injury?

7. How is a sibling's perspective of a head injured brother or sister different from that of a parent's?

8. What are the advantages and disadvantages of being a single parent coping with caregiver responsibilities?

(SET 11)

ENOUGH IS ENOUGH

Perspective: An often overlooked factor in addressing the needs of the person with a head trauma and their family is the impact of additional illnesses on the patient, other family members and/or primary caregivers. This can be a major issue because the resources of the support system can be greatly stressed. An example of this would be the following case overview:

Sandra was a 45 year old wife and mother of four children when she sustained a head injury. She had lived a very active, vigorous life and was the central figure in her family system. Caring for and managing Sandra was facilitated by the commitment of her husband, Vernon, who felt it was a privilege to care for his wife and best friend. Although their children were living in the same town, they were able to maintain their separate lives due to commitment and investment of their father. A major crisis occurred when their father suffered a severe heart attack and was in need of complete care himself. A temporary plan was to have an unmarried daughter move home to stabilize the situation. This worked for three weeks, until the daughter suffered a severe back injury while trying to lift her mother off of the floor.

Faced with a decision to either place the mother in a nursing home or have her move in with one of the children, the family was forced to realize that they had to become involved at a higher level of commitment and personal sacrifice. This decision never had to be made because both the mother and father died within one month. This case overview illustrates several points. First, a) viable caregiving arrangements can suddenly change, b) multiple illnesses can have a synergistic effect, overwhelm the resources of both caregiver and family.

Exploration:

1. Having read the above case synopsis, list other additional factors which could have further complicated this case.
2. Can you think of a family challenged by head injury that had to deal with the impact of multiple illnesses. a) What was the outcome? b) Were there any intergenerational issues? c) What would have been helpful.
3. What are some areas of competence that are important for families challenged by a head injury?
4. Who in your family would be able to shift roles and adapt to the changes caused by a head injury?
5. What are the assets and limitations of being involved with a self-help group?
6. Do you think that families can ever be normal again after a head injury?
7. Identify those extended family members who would not be helpful to you or your immediate family. State why.
8. If you are married, discuss how the severe head injury of your spouse would change and challenge your relationship. How would you treat your spouse? How would your spouse treat you? How has your spouse responded to prior crises and losses?
9. What are the major life problems your family has experienced?
10. Have these "problems" existed from generation to generation?
11. How does your family handle "bad news?"
12. What are the needs of your family that have never been met?
13. How much help would your family need to cope with a head injury?
14. How do you handle helplessness?
15. How does your family handle helplessness?
16. If your spouse was severely head injured, would you get a divorce?
17. If your spouse had AIDS, as well as a head injury what would you do? What would you need?

REFERENCES

Barker, L. (1988). Newsletter, 8(3), 2, National Head Injury Foundation, in E. A. Zeigler (1989), The importance of mutual support for spouses of head injury survivors. *Cognitive Rehabilitation, 7*(8), p.36.

Hart, T., & Jacobs, H. (1993). Rehabilitation and management of behavioral disturbances following frontal lobe injury. *Journal Head Trauma Rehabilitation, 8*(1), 1-12.

House, J. S. (1981). *Work stress and social support.* Reading, MA: Addison-Wesley.

Jacobs, H. E. (1984). *The family as a therapeutic agent: Long-term rehabilitation for traumatic head injury patients.* National Institute of Handicapped Research Report, Washington, D.C.

Keydel, C. F. (1991). *An exploration of perception and coping behavior in family members living with a closed head injured relative.* Unpublished doctoral dissertation, University of Maryland, College of Education, College Park.

Marmé, M., & Skord, K. (1993). Counseling strategies to enhance the vocational rehabilitation of persons after traumatic brain injury. *Journal of Applied Rehabilitation Counseling, 24*(1), 19-25.

Medlar, T. M. (1993). Sexual counseling and traumatic brain injury. *Sexuality and Disability, 11*(1), 57-71.

Sachs, P. R. (1991). *Treating families of brain injury survivors.* New York: Springer Publishing Company.

Treischmann, R. B. (1974). Coping with a disability: A sliding scale of goals. *Archives of Physical Medicine and Rehabilitation, 50,* 556-560.

Zeigler, E. A. (1989). The importance of mutual support for spouses of head injury survivors. *Cognitive Rehabilitation, 7*(3), 34-37.

7

The Crisis Of Head Injury In The Family:
A Helping Approach

7

THE CRISIS OF HEAD INJURY IN THE FAMILY: A HELPING APPROACH

When a family is impacted by head injury the health and human care professional is confronted by an event demanding the use of specific skills. For family members the crisis of head injury is not only stimulated by the trauma itself, but also by how they perceive the situation. Faced with a series of problems that appear to have no immediate solution, family members can become confused, extremely anxious, and can harbor feelings of intense helplessness. On the part of the family, initially, there may be the belief that they will be unable to deal with the trauma. Yet the crisis itself may not necessarily be only caused by the onset of the head injury event. Family crises can be precipitated by unexpected set-backs in the patient's recovery, behavior problems of siblings, the patient's cognitive and behavioral limitations which may cause episodic outbursts, and even the perceived unavailability of medical/treatment assistance (Hart & Jacobs, 1993; Orsillo, McCaffrey, & Fisher, 1993; Varney & Menefee, 1993). With head injury a family crisis may not be time-limited, nor may time be a healer of family emotions and thwarted expectations.

If head injury is responded to creatively and realistically by both health professionals and family members, the family's life can be more rewarding than it was before head injury; if not, the head injury experience can weaken the family and leave it more vulnerable to the stress of everyday problems. For the health care professional who is available to assist a family during the head injury crisis, effective intervention requires knowledge of what family members are experiencing emotionally during the event and skills to implement selected strategies. Since crisis also involves a sense of urgency and immediacy, an active approach must be used in order to relieve tension and counteract feelings of helplessness and hopelessness (Aquilera & Messick, 1974; Parad, 1965). The general goals of crisis intervention emphasize the here and now and include helping the family to restore itself to a state of equilibrium. In contrast to other goals of family treatment, and to the helping approach suggested in the previous chapter, helping a family in crisis involves short-term intervention which is directed both to alleviating the problem(s) that precipitated the crisis and to assisting the family to regain its ability to meet its own needs as it continues to adjust to the emerging reality of a disability (Epperson, 1977). Even with their attempts at continued adjustment, families are often faced with the joy of significant gain as well as the prolonged stress of limited progress.

A HELPING APPROACH

Many approaches have been suggested for working with families in crisis (Bard, 1973; Hafen & Peterson, 1982; Johnston, 1978; Rainsford & Schuman, 1981; Smith, 1978). But crisis intervention with the family, because of head injury trauma, can occur in three phases: the beginning phase, when there is the initial awareness of the trauma; a middle phase, when family members are becoming gradually aware of the extent of the trauma on both the patient and family life; and termination, when family members are energetically attempting to steady the unsteady state caused by the crisis. Each of these phases is relevant to varied forms of family crisis induced by the head injury. If the family's vulnerable state of equilibrium, for example, is upset by emotional outbursts, or dashed expectations, or a sudden financial emergency, then there will be an initial reaction, then a period when family members are aware of the impact of the crisis, and finally a time when the crisis is at least temporarily resolved. Each phase, moreover, varies in length, though frequently the crisis of head injury itself is long term, thus creating a situation of chronic crisis and long term need. Because of all the implications of head injury trauma on family life, many families appear to exist in a permanent state of "upset," going from one very tense situation to another.

BEGINNING PHASE

When the family is in crisis because of a head injury, the family members initially express fear, guilt, confusion, shock, and feelings of vulnerability. Blame may exist between family members, and the family may express distorted expectations for the patient. Family members may constantly ask themselves the question: "Why?"

At this time, the family primarily needs emotional support, to focus on the present, and to begin to understand their own perceptions of the meaning of what has happened. Before family members can begin to attend to the present and to express their own beliefs about what they perceive is the "crisis" for the family, they need someone just to be with them to attend, to listen, and to respond to their feelings. Gradually, the family members will want to talk about how this crisis has affected them and the patient, but are more willing to do so when they are convinced that the health professional wishes to listen and to share their grief, hope, anger, and disappointment. Listening and acknowledging the legitimacy of family feelings can communicate confidence to the family, and on their part, trust in the helping professional. During their initial reaction to the crisis, family members usually want to ventilate their feelings and need empathy and understanding. When listening, health care professionals can begin to learn how the family understands the crisis, and importantly, its cause. The identification of the particular stressors within family life, as well as specific family needs, should be accomplished, however, in the context of continued emotional support.

Once this atmosphere of acceptance and trust has been established, then the health care professional can assist the family to explore actively all the reality issues resulting from the crisis, such as financial implications, change in family role responsibilities, and modification of treatment and/or management plans. The health care professional will also need to understand what adaptive mechanisms are already operating in the family and how the family has coped with past crises (Jacobson, 1980). Often the problem itself that has precipitated the crisis can be "broken down" into manageable pieces, and each aspect of the problem is then dealt with by family members.

With the provision of support, the identification of what is needed to restore family equilibrium, the ventilation of family feelings surrounding the crisis event, and the realization by family members that someone cares, intervention goals are gradually formulated as the health care professional begins to understand the meaning head injury has for the family. The health care professional should be careful not to give false reassurances, but to make contact with the family at the family's level of reality. Some families may be too overwhelmed with the realistic problems caused by the crisis to have any energy immediately available for expressing grief. The expression of feelings may follow the temporary resolution of such practical difficulties as finances and patient management demands.

MIDDLE PHASE

As the family members gradually gain an understanding of the crisis, and face the reality of what has happened, they will begin to ask such questions as: "What can we do to help the person with a head injury ... How can we manage this disruption to our family life?" Feelings of anger, guilt, self-pity, disappointment, sadness, and loss will still continue, but family members begin to search for answers and to explore what are the best ways to cope with this family "upset." The family's search for answers may demand a specific response, but many questions will have no answer. There may be no discernible reason why either the head injury has occurred, or for the existence of the present crisis, but the reality is that it has occurred and if the family and the patient are to survive, then the crisis must be addressed. The bottom line may be that life is not fair, but family needs must be attended to as the family gradually takes responsibility for resolving, as much as possible as it can be resolved, the present crisis.

As the health care professional understands that the family is slowly coming to grips with the meaning of what has happened, at the same time the professional needs to recognize that family members will continue to express their feelings about the crisis, and this expression may take many forms. For example, anger may be expressed as passive resistance, sarcasm, or ridicule of persons on whom the patient or family depends. Frequently, the health professional will become the target of anger. When this happens, one should assist family members to identify the origin of these feelings and how they are related to the crisis situation. With anger, family members may also deny any of the implications of what has happened, such as permanent loss to cognitive or physical functions. This denial may be necessary in order to give the family members time to marshal their resources and cope with an unacceptable reality.

During this intervention state, the health care professional continues to listen, and encourages the family members to understand not only the possible problem areas for adjustment, but also their own internal and external resources that can be utilized to deal with the crisis. Prior, coping strategies and a network of established friends and family for support are valuable resources in times of crisis. With this encouragement, moreover, the concerned and skilled professional can stimulate the family to enter into a dialogue in which mutual feelings can be recognized and different solutions can be shared to the varied problems emerging from the crisis.

As the family begins to understand more fully the meaning of head injury to family life, certain tasks related to family reorganization may then be assigned. These duties may involve contacting, when possible, the extended family, performing other chores in the home, or using designated community supports such as local chapters of the National Head Injury Foundation as well as other resources (Appendices A and B). Yet the health care professional should be aware of the separate needs of each family member and what is the most difficult struggle for each person in the family. These may vary from the children who want to spend more time in the hospital with a sibling to parents who may wonder how they are going to care for a head injured child after they are divorced. As family members communicate more with each other about their own needs, then family reorganization is handled more easily.

The main goal of this phase is to assist the family to begin to adapt to the reality of the crisis. It involves helping the family move from a state of perceived helplessness, confusion, and disorientation to an emotional level where these feelings are minimized and such additional feelings as anger, guilt, and blame begin to be controlled.

TERMINATION PHASE

When the health care professional realizes that family equilibrium is being restored, adjustment problems are being addressed and family members are involved in many of the solutions to problems emanating from the crisis, then contact with the family may well depend on the changing needs related to the head injury process. Continued contact from the health care professional will usually be necessary. Given the frequent long term nature of severe head injury, and the different crises that can unexpectedly occur, most families need long term support. The terminating phase is more of a journey than a destination.

CONCLUSION

During the head injury crisis intervention, health care professionals have multiple functions. As an assessor, they try to determine how the head injury experience affects the entire family, as well as consider the possibility that emotional symptoms may be related to a previous family crisis. The situation is evaluated as adequately and thoroughly as possible, and the health and human care professional learns about the total situation of the family and how they can develop, when necessary, effective problem-solving skills. The health care professional is also a resource person, providing information about: a) head injury and its implications for family life, b) the resources available in the community for the family, c) how family roles can be readjusted to accommodate the new, caring needs of the patient, and d) how the extended family or kin network can be developed as a resource. Because the family members should recognize their feelings and attitudes related to head injury, the health care professional is a facilitator for the expression of these feelings, as well as a source of support by listening and reinforcing the collective strengths of the family. At this time the reality of head injury cannot be eradicated but its impact can, should and must be made more bearable for all involved.

The following personal statement, "Life Is Never Uncomplicated," by Keith Smith, explores the long, complex and challenging journey of a young man who is committed to living his life to the fullest.

Personal Statement

LIFE IS NEVER UNCOMPLICATED
by Keith Smith

In 1982, I was a junior at a state university. I was studying psychology and bartending at a local country club. My life was average and there were no complications. Then, while I was riding my motorcycle home from a date, I was hit by a drunk driver. Fortunately, I was wearing a helmet. This reduced but did not prevent the closed head injury I experienced that has changed my life. I also experienced other physical injuries that have also influenced my life since this 'accident' some 11 years ago.

After eight days in a coma, I awoke in the intensive care unit of a local hospital. I don't remember much from the first few months except confusion and being in traction (for my fractured femur). I was very fortunate during these days. I received continuous support from my family and friends. Despite their shock, my parents visited me everyday, my friends weekly. Their influence helped me begin to reorient to reality and my previous life, things I did not have a very good grasp on in the early months.

Initially I was unable to recognize the important people in my life. Eventually I began to recognize these people as my family and friends. My parents received support from their friends through these difficult times. Also, early on, they were contacted by a speech therapist associated with a local rehabilitation center. She assisted them in understanding my injuries and planning my rehabilitation. With her assistance my parents were able to arrange my admission to a rehabilitation center located in another state. There I began what I consider my true rehabilitation and recovery.

I entered this rehabilitation center about three months after my injury. My physical injuries and my parents' uncertainty about being able to control me necessitated the usage of an ambulance. A close friend of mine accompanied us on this journey. It is at this point that my memories become clear; I remember the ambulance trip and my admission to the hospital.

I was quite frightened when my parents left me at this strange place ... I cried and begged them not leave me there. I finally became convinced that I would only reside there for a short time and accepted being there. I was convinced that the reason that I was there was because of my physical injuries; I did not believe that there was anything wrong with my brain. I was unaware of the disorders in my thought process. I was convinced that when I overcame my physical injuries I would be back in school. Having had less serious physical injuries when I was younger, I was sure that I could overcome these injuries as I had overcome the ones from my past. The concept of brain injury was foreign to me.

At the rehabilitation hospital, I experienced physical, psychological and cognitive therapy. Shortly after I began my work there,

I began to realize that my thinking was impaired. This realization created a determination in me to overcome the impairments in my thinking. This decision was probably the most critical one that I have ever made. Even now, the drive to overcome my mental difficulties continues. Now with a purpose, I requested and received as much therapy as I could take. Part of these efforts included an urge to better understand my brain and what had happened to me. Combined with this was the continued support of my friends and family. I don't believe that I could have done as well as I have without that. They helped me believe that there was still a place in the world for me, despite my disabilities. This was very important since during this initial rehabilitation I felt pretty worthless.

After several months at this hospital, a frustrating situation to be certain, I went home. When I reached home, I was more physically and spiritually fit as well as being glad to be home. I still had impairments, but really believed that I had overcome most of them. I even thought that I understood my cognitive difficulties. After all, since I had learned a "bunch" of terms to describe them, didn't that mean I had control of them? Of course I was being unrealistic; knowing the words did not solve the problems I had yet to face.

It was at home I learned what it really means to be disabled. My physical disabilities were easily understood by the people that knew me; it was the mental ones that they did not understand. I was frustrated by their lack of understanding, especially since I could explain it to them. I always talked in the past tense as if I was not still impaired. I didn't realize that these 'explanations' merely emphasized that I was still impaired. It was then that I learned who my true friends really were. I felt a lot of pain as I lost some of them and my belief in myself began to lower. What had happened to the friends that had been so supportive earlier? Why didn't I see them any more? I was even more unsure of myself at this point; I wasn't so sure that I could ever be 'normal' again. Fortunately, while I lost a number of friends, others stayed with me and tried to help me. It did not seem to matter to them that I had a poor memory and only talked about my injuries and nothing else. A couple of the people that I had grown up with stuck it out. In fact, they made efforts to bring back memories of my past that I had lost. The support that they gave to me through the hard times creates a debt that I feel that I can never repay. Because of them I remember things that would have otherwise have been lost. One of the people who did not stay with me was my girlfriend. I was quite hurt by this, and it made me more shy and afraid to even consider approaching a woman for a date. In fact, my low self-esteem made it difficult to make new friends with anyone.

All of this was going on as I went to physical and cognitive therapy several days a week. Since I believed that I had pretty much overcome the cognitive deficits, the physical therapy was more understandable than the cognitive. That is, until one day when I suddenly realized that there was another, better way of solving the problem that I was working on in cognitive therapy. I was shocked!

The idea that I had not really overcome the brain injury threw me for a loop. Then I remembered my resolution to overcome all of the effects of my brain injury. That drive was still there, and I became a very cooperative client, striving to understand and do better. From that point on, the cognitive therapy became as important to me as the physical therapy. One of the consequences of this attitude, besides driving me to achieve, was the creation of an attitude about the quality of my work; I became a perfectionist. The perfectionist attitude about my work both helped and hindered me as life went on. It drove me to achieve, and it made me view anything but a perfect score or an "A" as unsatisfactory, a failure. This created overreactions to my failures at anything. It also set me up for depression since no one can do everything perfectly. It is only years later after much work with my psychologist that I have adopted a more reasonable attitude, such as doing things as well as I can, but not having an unrealistic expectation of doing everything perfectly, and being satisfied that at least I tried the best I could.

It was during my work in rehabilitation that I began to prepare to re-enter college. Despite my difficulties, I was still convinced that I could eventually become a psychologist. The first course that I took was a repeat of a course that I had already taken. In this first attempt, I did not do as well as I had originally done. This was extremely frustrating since I had received a "B" when I originally taken it. It also demonstrated to me that there were still impairments that I had not overcome. For example, I could not get by in my courses as I previously had done. I began to think that some other types of efforts than the ones that I had used before would be required to achieve what I wanted. It was also at this point that my therapists began to suggest that I reconsider the direction that I was taking. The suggested that I consider a career in another field. I ignored these suggestions; I was convinced that if I really tried, I could achieve the goals that I set for myself before my injuries. I believed that I could overcome my cognitive impairments, as I had done with the physical ones, or at least learned how to compensate. I took this attitude even though I still had difficulties with attention, concentration and memory. Since I had my job back as assistant head bartender and was doing fine, what could stop me now? Despite this external positive attitude, I knew I was brain injured. I figure, with assistance, that I might be making a mistake betting everything on this major. After all, I did have impaired thinking so I began to consider hedging my bet. I decided that after I took a couple of semesters I would reconsider my major, but not yet. At least, that was what I told them. I never believed that I would not be able to obtain my major, psychology, if for no reason other than to prove them wrong.

In my first enrolled regular semester, a year after my injury, I took two senior level laboratory courses. I also began to assist in an experiment being run by one of the professors. I realized quickly that I had overextended myself so I dropped one of the lab courses. Then came the first test. The grade that I received was the lowest in the class despite my efforts and interest. I was shocked. This was not me, I don't fail exams! Maybe they were right since apparently I could not deal with the abstract reasoning this profession required, maybe I should change majors. If I had completed that semester, I would have certainly failed that course. But during that semester, the first real setback that I had experienced since my injury occurred when it was discovered that I had a 90% hearing loss in one of my ears. This was due to an infection in the middle ear which destroyed most of the bones that transmit sound. During the corrective surgery, it was discovered that the infection had spread to the brain. I required a craniotomy to correct this, and I was once again in intensive care. I was quite upset, even panicked. Fortunately, I did not have much time to consider this second head trauma. The unfairness of it struck me. I wasn't sure if the efforts that I had been making were really worth it. Well, I survived the operation and received the good news that it was not malignant, so I figured that I could go on with my life with some new scars.

Two days after I got home from the hospital, I was back in the hospital again. I had developed a seizure disorder from the surgery and had had a seizure, a disorder that I will never overcome even though I control it with an anticonvulsive. I became extremely upset from this new setback, I thought my life was over. I had a million questions. Why me? Why do I have to have this additional difference from normal? I overreacted to this new complication. I felt that I would be more impaired by this disorder than I actually am. I really thought that my life was over. I even began to consider that one-way path–suicide. I did not know that millions of people are able to live with epilepsy and seizure disorders. It was only through extensive counseling that I was able to accept my seizure disorder.

In the following ten years since I developed this disease, I have had two seizures. I am always hospitalized for about a week after these seizures, and there is always an insufficient level of the anticonvulsent in my system and/or excessive stress in my life. Now, when things become difficult, I take tranquilizers or antidepressants to help stabilize my emotions and prevent them from reoccurring. Now I never miss a dose of my anticonvulsent medication or drink alcohol.

After my first semester and my surgery and seizure, I signed up for my second semester, which I completed. In my undergraduate career after my injury, I never took more than three courses in a semester and received mainly B's. I had learned ways to compensate for my difficulties. Even though I never felt that I was like the other students and I spent two or three times as much time on the course work as they did, I was able to complete my Bachelor of Science degree in Psychology. I had the greatest difficulty with courses that required a great deal of memory, like human anatomy. These courses I took several times, auditing them first, then taking them for credit. As I passed more and more courses, my self-esteem increased. The idea that I might not be able to complete a degree in this field faded away as the course work became easier and easier as time passed. The day that I finally walked across the stage to receive my degree was the proudest day in my life. I had done it; I had proven them wrong and obtained that degree just as I had planned before I was injured. I knew then that I had overcome the injury that I had received some eight years earlier.

Several important events occurred during my undergraduate career that bear mentioning.

Some two years after my injury, I won a personal injury suit against the person that had hit me. I won this suit because it appeared that I would not be able to continue the career that I had aimed at. Winning the settlement created a dilemma for me. Should I continue the difficulties that I was having in school and continue to prove them wrong, or should I just relax? I had already proven some of the doctors wrong, but how could I stop now? I took some time off and soon realized that without the challenges created by school, I was bored. Besides, how could I stop that drive I have to overcome my difficulties. So I moved out, my first true independence since the injury, and re-enrolled in school. Of course having money made me different from most students in still another way. This was easier to overcome than the other more obvious consequences of my injuries, especially the seizures. So, I kept my mouth shut and didn't always drive my sports car; I tried to appear like an average student.

The other major event during my undergraduate career occurred some four years after my injury. I became a peer counselor at a new rehabilitation facility that worked with head-injured adults. My psychologist, whom I continue to see, suggested it, and supervised my work at the facility. This was a true learning experience. I learned how to assist others who had experienced injuries similar to my own. These improvements in my interpersonal skills generalized out to my personal life. Before I began this experience, I had neither the confidence nor the skills to ask a woman for a date. These deficits had prevented me from asking anyone out despite my psychologist's and friend's encouragement. Sometime after I started at this facility, I began the first interpersonal relationship since my injury. I learned from that experience how vulnerable I was to my emotions. I had not control over them. I had some difficulties relating to this person, not recognizing the cues that people give to each other in interpersonal relations. It did allow me to practice my new interpersonal skills. I learned that others would accept me despite my deficits. I also learned that others also had some difficulties in college, and that I really had no deficits, at least ones that showed when I dealt with other people. In fact, other than maybe mentioning the seizure disorder, I did not have to say anything about my disabilities. Since I realized that I had really overcome many of the ones that I had had, I was very much like a normal person.

After I received my degree, I continued my work as a peer counselor as I tried to determine what I would do next. I had received my degree in psychology, but I did not have a grade point average high enough to get into one of the area schools. I did not want to leave the area; I had all of my doctors, my family and my friends in the area. So, in order to keep my college skills up, I took a summer school course in rehabilitation counseling. The instructor of that course was the head of the rehabilitation counseling department at the university. After several discussion with him, I decided to apply. I was fairly uncertain about trying to get into graduate school, as it involved taking the Miller Analogies Exam. Exams of that type have always been difficult for me, but now I had a challenge, getting into the graduate program. I studied hard and obtained a sufficient grade to allow me to enroll in the master's program in rehabilitation counseling.

I found graduate school easier in some ways than the undergraduate program. The program was structured, taught material that was directive and had more meaning than the general information taught in undergraduate studies. Well, I was very proud of myself. I have been able to maintain an A average in all of my course work. Since I began there has been only one setback. About one year after I started, I developed a toxic reaction to my anticonvulsent. Because of this, I was unable to complete a semester. In fact, I lost almost a year because of this difficulty. I completed the courses that I had not finished. In fact, now as I write this, I have almost completed my master's degree in Rehabilitation Counseling, and I am a therapist at a rehabilitation center. Through the years, from when I first became aware enough to understand what had happened to me, I have grown in many ways. It is almost like I was reborn when I was first injured. Although the growth is slower now than when I started, it has not stopped.

DISCUSSION QUESTIONS ON THE PERSONAL STATEMENT
"LIFE IS NEVER UNCOMPLICATED"

1. How does an uncomplicated life prior to head injury help or hinder the adjustment process?

2. Does the potential of reducing a head injury justify a law requiring the wearing of a helmet?

3. How can the "terror" of "leaving" a family member at a hospital or rehabilitation facility be made more bearable?

4. Does a history of having overcome prior injuries help or hinder the adjustment to a head injury?

5. What are the advantages and disadvantages of being unaware of the extent of your head injury?

6. How can lack of awareness of limitations create stress for the family?

7. In this personal statement, the importance of support from family and friends is stressed. How would you develop a support system for those persons who do not have family or friends?

8. What does Keith mean by being physically and spiritually fit?

9. Why are "mental" disabilities more complicated than physical disabilities?

10. Can the drive to overcome a limitation be a source of frustration and disappointment?

11. Why was it difficult for Keith to accept the changes in his life?

12. Discuss the stress created by the craniotomy. Why did Keith feel it was unfair?

13. Why was the epilepsy so problematic for Keith?

14. What were the stressors created by winning the personal injury suit?

15. Why was it difficult for Keith to negotiate an interpersonal relationship?

16. What did Keith mean by, "being like a normal person" and "being reborn"?

(SET 12)

FRAGILE: HANDLE WITH CARE

Perspective: When families are forced by reality to address the complexity and permanence of a head injury, there is an urgent need for them to be listened to, appreciated, valued and understood.

By listening, caring and responding, the family is validated and given the opportunity to establish a communication process that is based upon real issues, mutual respect and hope, based upon reality and not desperation.

Exploration:
1. Develop a list of what you need to maintain a sense of well being and a positive quality of life.
   a.
   b.
   c.
   d.
   e.
   f.

     g.
     h.
     i.
     j.

2. Develop a list of what you need or would need to help you negotiate the stress of a the head injury experience.
     a.
     b.
     c.
     d.
     e.
     f.
     g.
     h.
     i.
     j.

3. What should health care professionals be taught in school regarding the needs of persons and families challenged by a head injury?

4. How could religious organizations expand their role in helping families to cope with long-term illnesses and disabilities in general and head injury in particular?

5. What would you and your family expect from the medical-rehabilitation team in the treatment of a family member with a head injury?

6. How would you want your employer to treat you if you sustained a head injury on the job? How would you be treated?

7. How would you respond if you "caused" the head injury of your child and your spouse blamed you and wanted a divorce?

8. How have you and your family been treated by medical and rehabilitation personnel?

9. Have you ever experienced non-helpful behavior?

10. What was most helpful to you and your family when you experienced a medical crisis?

11. From your personal or professional frame of reference, develop a list of management techniques you have found to be helpful or not helpful in working with the person having a head injury.

HELPFUL - WHY NOT HELPFUL - WHY NOT
     a.
     b.
     c.
     d.
     e.
     f.
     g.

REFERENCES

Aquilera, D. C., & Messick, J. M. (1974). *Crisis intervention: Theory and methodology* (2nd ed.). St. Louis: C.V. Mosby, Co.

Bard, M. (1973). *Family crisis intervention: From concept to implementation*. U.S. Department of Justice, Washington, D.C.

Epperson, M. M. (1977). Families in sudden crisis. *Social Work in Health Care, 2*(3), 265-273.

Hafen, B. Q., & Peterson, B. (1982). *The crisis intervention handbook*. Englewood Cliffs, New Jersey: Prentice-Hall, Inc.

Hart, T., & Jacobs, H. (1993). Rehabilitation and management of behavioral disturbances following frontal lobe injury. *Journal Head Trauma Rehabilitation, 8*(1), 1-12.

Jacobson, G. F. (1980). Crisis theory. In G. F. Jacobson (Ed.), *Crisis intervention in the 1980s* (pp.52-72). San Francisco: Jossey-Bass.

Johnston, D. C. (1978). Crisis intervention skills. *Journal of Practical Nursing*, 16-19.

Orsillo, S. M., McCaffrey, R. J., & Fisher, J. M. (1993). Siblings of head-injured individuals: A population at risk. *Journal Head Trauma Rehabilitation, 8*(1), 102-115.

Parad, H. (1965). *Crisis intervention: Selected readings*. New York: Family Service Association of America.

Rainsford, G. L., & Schuman, S. H. (1981). The family in crisis. *Journal of the American Medical Association, 256*, 60-63.

Smith, L. L. (1978, July). A review of crisis intervention theory. *Social Casework*, pp. 396-405.

Varney, W. R., & Meneffe, L. (1993). Psychosocial and executive deficits following closed head injury: Implications for orbital frontal cortex. *Journal Head Trauma Rehabilitation, 8*(1), 32-44.

8

Loss, Grief, and Head Injury

8

LOSS, GRIEF, AND HEAD INJURY

The existence of a head injury will not only cause a crisis in family life, but may also cause a family to enter a state of grief that is intense and enduring. Family crises are usually temporary and are characterized by anxiety and a searching for immediate solutions. However, when a family is challenged by head injury, the feelings of resentment, anger, and sadness resulting from patient and family losses can linger and cause a serious disruption to family functioning. With the family's bereavement consequent to head injury, emphasis is not necessarily on the immediate resolution of the grief but on assisting the family members to function effectively as they gradually manage their own sorrow. This management and possible alleviation of grief require certain specialized skills.

Grief is a family experience of coping with the loss of what was as it clashes with the current reality of the family and the person impacted by a head injury. Grief responses by family members include emotions, thoughts, and behaviors which occur as a reaction to perceived family losses (Kane, 1990). Many losses are significant chiefly because of their symbolic meaning (Brown, 1990). The perception of the importance of what has been lost affects the intensity and the duration of the grief. Yet grief is a normal and healthy reaction to loss, though the strength and the duration of the family's grief response is not predictable. Kane (1990) believes that readjustment to loss and the achievement of positive change is dependent on one's coping capabilities, the family members' flexibility and adaptability, internalized locus of control, and adaptive skills. For the family expressing grief, intervention efforts are not so much directed to alleviating the immediate pain but to increasing the ability of the family member to change appropriately with the loss.

The abilities to listen, respond, provide support, impart information, and facilitate the family exchange of feeling are needed by health care professionals to assist families in coping with intense grief. To help families to cope with loss also requires specific knowledge of the family, how its members handle grief, and the ability to apply this understanding at times when family emotions are intense. Often those family members who adjust to the loss do so by drawing upon their resources and find new meaning in living in spite of their family structure, dreams, and resources having been greatly altered. This point is addressed by McKinlay and Hickox (1988) when they state:

> ... severe head injury may involve a loss of important qualities
> that were part of the person's premorbid personality. As with a
> true bereavement, role changes are often necessary (p.71).

Although the topics of death and dying are usually associated with bereavement, head injury is an event that can cause family grief because it emerges from a pervasive sense of loss. The family's eventual realization that their family member will never be the same person and that family life is now very different can cause lingering feelings of deep sorrow. In contrast to a family crisis, which can be temporary or at least minimized through problem solving strategies, family loss and bereavement represent constant companions to family life. The grief, though diminished in its intensity with the passage of time, can be a pervading theme in family life.

Because loss and grief management provoke different intervention strategies, this chapter suggests a helping approach to assist families in bereavement related to head injury. Three areas are emphasized: 1) general considerations to be aware of when helping a family impacted by head injury; 2) obstacles to effective grieving, and 3) interventions focused on meeting the family's needs.

GENERAL CONSIDERATIONS

Before beginning intervention with a bereaved family, the health care professional should reflect upon certain factors, an understanding of which will facilitate an effective helping approach that is relevant to the family living a head injury experience.

1. **Knowing Yourself As A Health Care Professional.**
   During bereavement, some family members may become extremely distraught. At these times, the health care professional may feel helpless, anxious, fearful, and may become emotionally distressed. To experience anxiety and discomfort is normal, but these feelings can become so intense that they can hinder any helping efforts. In assisting the bereaved family there is always going to be some agony, but if health care professionals have an insight into their own defenses against grief and pain, then many feelings of discomfort can be controlled.

2. **Understanding The Stages Of The Grief Process.**
    Professional literature reports several descriptive models of the
    grief response (Bowlby, 1961; Brown & Stoudemine, 1983;
    Kubler-Ross, 1969). Kane (1990) identifies a four-stage process of
    grief as a response to loss. In this theory, grief resolution is an
    unchanging succession, and the activities of a stage are the ideas,
    emotions, and behaviors particular to it. These stages are (1)
    ignoring the loss, (2) experiencing the loss, (3) understanding the
    loss, and (4) changing with the loss.

    Matz (1978) has developed a more lengthy descriptive model
    which captures many of the family's behavioral reactions,
    although families may differ in how they react to the loss. Matz
    believes that there are different stages of mourning in response
    to a traumatic event, and if a bereaved family is to reach an
    adaptive stage, then family members will usually follow predict-
    able steps in their grieving process. The stages are: 1) "If I deny
    it, it's not true." The first response to a serious loss is usually
    denial, although Matz believes that the denial stage is "punctu-
    ated" by times of painful emotional awareness. The denial helps
    the family members to function and meet many of their daily
    responsibilities. 2) "I have the power to undo it." The denial
    gradually gives way to feelings of omnipotence. These feelings
    may be characterized by attempting to bring back the loss, by
    searching efforts, or may be expressed as anger at events or
    people the bereaved family regards as responsible for the loss.
    Unfortunately these efforts are doomed to fail, and gradually
    despair and helplessness occur. 3) "I can't do anything about it."
    Matz explains this is a time when the bereaved family members
    face the loss and begin to understand their feelings in order to
    reach an adaptive solution. The past may be reexamined,
    perhaps given up and partially replaced with hope. Depression
    also occurs, but hope may overcome it. 4) "I am rebuilding and
    every now and then I remember." The bereaved family members
    start to rebuild their lives. Social patterns are reestablished and
    new decisions are made to reach personal and family goals.
    According to Matz, painful memories will arise, but the family
    members appear to have more strength to deal with these
    emotions. With all of these steps, however, the phases them-
    selves do not have clear-cut beginnings and endings. The move
    from phase to phase is a gradual process rather than sudden and
    dramatic.

3. **Understanding Intense Grief Reaction.** Intervention
    approaches will differ between the family that has become very
    dysfunctional consequent to the losses associated with the head
    injury experience and the family that is still attempting to
    maintain its balance and perspective. For example, when family
    members deny the loss, are evasive in their communication,

show an absence of basic self-care as well as nurturance, and have persistent anger, guilt, hopelessness, and depression, they are displaying very serious adjustment problems. In contrast, the family that is expressing an appropriate reactive sadness has begun to confront the reality of the head injury and is able to meet its responsibilities. Family communication styles are still intact. There may be some regression by the family members to more childish, aggressive behaviors, but this is temporary. Their sadness is actually a necessary part of the grieving process and the help provided to the family is mainly directed toward providing support for the alleviation of grief feelings and providing role models.

4. **Understanding The Concepts of Centrality, Peripheral, Preventable, and Unpreventable.** Bugen (1977) explains the meaning of these terms as follows: if the person is central to family life such as a loving parent or successful child, the loss will be greater than that associated with a person who is peripheral to the family. Whether the trauma was preventable or unpreventable will influence both anger and blame associated with the intensity of the loss response. All these terms are important to understand because the health care professional frequently assists the family to move from a belief in preventability to a belief in unpreventability. If the person is central and the family members are convinced it was preventable, then, as Bugen states, the grief will be both intense and prolonged. Initial intervention with the family will entail an assessment of the relationship of the impact of head injury to the expectations, values, and beliefs of the family members.

5. **Understanding the Flexibility of Goals for the Family Challenged by a Head Injury.** Families who are experiencing head injury will have different needs. Many family members are looking for some alleviation of the feelings of loneliness and depression, whereas others are searching for a way to integrate the loss into family life. The challenge for families is to accept the loss, adapt to the loss, and try to assimilate the chronic sorrow into the family system. The harsh reality is that certain events of the life experience must be accepted for what they are and not what we want them to be.

OBSTACLES TO PROGRESS IN GRIEVING

With these considerations that represent areas of understanding for intervention in family loss, there are specific roadblocks to effective grieving. Brown (1990) has identified these barriers as:

1. Persistent denial of the permanent cognitive and physical losses. Family members continuously talk about "what was," and the past is continually reviewed or dwelled upon in order to maintain hopes for full recovery and restoration of function.

2. Inability to express negative affect because of the loss. Bowlby (1973) explains that anger and crying are necessary responses that can lead to the recognition that the loss is final. The inability to cry or rave at the loss is often a consequence of society's dictates to maintain appropriate composure at the actual time of the loss. Or, the initial grief response may be inhibited because of the family member's fear of how a grief reaction may affect the injured family member, or other family members. Some families may even believe that the release of angry feelings associated with a loss is inappropriate.

3. Difficulties in dealing with ambivalence and feelings of resentment related to the loss. Brown (1990) reports that the closer and more positive the relationship with the lost object, the more difficult and prolonged the grief reaction can be.

4. Unfinished business related to other losses. The current losses resulting from the head trauma may stimulate previously unresolved grief related to past losses that have never been completely resolved.

5. Absence of limited coping skills or support network. Many family members may not possess adequate coping skills that can be accessed at the time of loss.

An Intervention Approach

Intervention should begin as soon as possible after the occurrence of a head injury. Yet this is dependent upon the family's needs and their ability to respond. Loss and bereavement adaptation is both a healing and a rebuilding process, and a timetable cannot be set (Kane, 1990).

In assisting a family challenged by head injury, it is important for the members to understand the source of their loss, then admit this loss and express their fear as well as their hope. The intervention goal does not have to be family rebuilding but rather stabilization of the family so the rebuilding process can begin when appropriate.

The first meeting with the family, whether in the hospital, a clinic, an office, or the family home, is vitally important. It sets the tone for the remaining family contacts. For example, if the initial family encounter is characterized by the health care professional's questions and an explanation of head injury, then the remaining family counseling will be a procedural explanation, almost an intellectual exercise, and not tap the emotions underlying the family's reaction to head injury. On the other hand, if, during the family visit, the health care professional assumes the role of a listener, a facilitator for the expression of feelings, and begins to understand family dynamics, then the remaining family visits and/or interventions will help the family members to understand their grief. However, information at this point can be helpful if it is presented at a level that is congruent with individual family needs.

During this first meeting, and as family members attempt to experience and perhaps understand their own grief, good listening is shown by communicating a sense of caring, attending to the present family concerns, suspending judgements, and not attempting to compare the health care professional's experience with the family's experience. Kane (1990) believes that effective helping with grief includes "maintaining a presence with the griever rather than solve the griever's problems ... not by attempting to remove the griever's pain, but instead, by allowing the griever to feel the pain of the loss." (p.221). Active listening can help the family because it communicates an acceptance of the family and invites the family members to share their worries and anxieties. Active listening also promotes the opportunity for family members to express themselves, namely, perhaps to moan and complain without others' criticism. A response such as "This is normal" is frequently the most reassuring information for the family. The expression of family feelings is further encouraged when the helper reflects their emotions by such statements as "You are upset because ... you must be disappointed because ..." This reflection is not intended to operate at deep emotional levels but is a paraphrase of what has been said (Anthony & Carkhuff, 1976).

In the beginning family meetings, the health care professional should learn what the family understands about why the loss occurred, the effectiveness of the informal and formal supportive systems available to the family, and the family members' ability to cope effectively with stress. How an individual adapts after loss is generally determined by one's individual coping skills. Matz (1978) has identified these goals as the determinants of successful grief resolution. The family must become aware of the basic source of the loss, because what may be perceived by the health care professional as the cause of family grief may only be another symptom of a more serious problem. For example, the occurrence of a head injury for a parent who has a long family history of alcoholism and being away from home for prolonged periods may renew feelings of resentment, especially if that person has undergone alcoholism rehabilitation before the diagnosis. Family members may still harbor deep emotions about the patient's earlier behavior. This represents "unfinished business," and the new diagnosis aggravates these feelings because it symbolizes another source of unpleasantness for the family.

During these family visits, it may be necessary for family members to review past events, and perhaps to repeat going over the past, for this expression can help family members to verbalize their feelings and then eventually make sense out of the loss. The family must ask the unanswerable "whys" over and over again before adjustment to the loss can take place. Piece by piece, the links with the past are re-examined, grieved over, given up, and partially replaced with the hope that what is lost may be compensated for or even replaced by another source of personal or family satisfaction.

As family members review the past and express their feelings about the loss in a non-judgemental context, as they begin to understand the meaning and implications of the loss to family life, they are then making adaptive progress to a loss resolution. Adjustment to the loss involves change, a change from perhaps the old ways at managing family responsibilities to a different outlook for the future, to modifications in the family duties, and even to making new choices for their own future. Slowly, the family may adjust to the implications of the new situation resulting from the head trauma. The health care professional can often facilitate this change by sharing one's own feelings over the necessity to choose in an uncertain situation, engaging in relevant and personal disclosure, and challenging the family members to identify the advantages from making any changes that result in loss adaptation. Family members should be very active in the process as they search for new meaning and purpose while living with the head injury trauma.

When the health care professional has determined that the family members have a better understanding of the source of the loss, their reaction to it, and how adjustment could be achieved, and also believes that a trusting relationship has been established with the family members, then a course of action to meet the adjustment goals can be planned. The plan of action may take many forms, namely, providing support, reassurance, role models, information to help the family members move through the grief stages, and/or utilizing situational supports and resources. Grief resolution is encouraged by having a variety of well-integrated resources available to a family. Pastoral care, neighborhood crisis clinics, and friends can provide valuable assistance during the bereavement period. Identifying with others through support groups often helps both towards acceptance of the loss and acknowledgment that changes should be made in family life. Also, contact with the local chapter of The National Head Injury Foundation and other resources can be helpful (see Appendix A and B).

The information imparted to a family should focus on more than the losses associated with head injury. Although the loss may become temporarily the most striking feature of family life, the remaining resource opportunities could be emphasized. These resources are often the established family strengths or environmental supports readily available to family members. Also, providing information may frequently mean reinforcing health care knowledge, suggesting new expectations for the family members, or reviving expectations for each other that might have been lost at the onset of the head injury. Through this information exchange process the health care professional assists the family members both to become aware of each other's needs and to learn how to use the networks of support both within and outside of the home. The goal is to keep the family intact, and to help them to realize that "life can be worth living" during and after the head injury experience. By supporting the learning of new information and skills, while attending to each other's needs and expressing feelings, the family can begin the process of rebuilding, refocusing and rejuvenating. However, this perspective is based upon the awareness that surviving and living beyond the trauma of a head injury is hard work!

During this time of intervention, the family assumes the responsibility for any needed change. With the bereaved family there may be a terminating phase, but the members usually want the opportunity for periodic dialogue with the initial health care professional during the years that characterize adjustment to head injury. They may want someone they can turn to when the painful reality of the loss occasionally becomes overwhelming. Consequently, contact with the family is important until it is mutually perceived that the family is coping successfully and does not need or desire further involvement with the health care professional. This is where self help groups have a significant role to play because they are often more understanding and available to the person with head injury and their family throughout the life span (see Appendix A).

CONCLUSION

The occurrence of a family loss related to head injury is a powerful, encompassing and dynamic experience. In order for family members to cope effectively they often need skillful and relevant intervention. They need someone who can be there to listen, to offer reassurance, and to validate their feelings. For the family living with the reality of head injury, intervention can take many forms but it is always guided by the conviction that underlying all approaches is the willingness to share another's loss as well as hopes and dreams. Such sharing is frequently the beginning of a resolution of the family loss and recognition that life is livable even though it will never be the same.

The following personal statement, "For Better or For Worse," by David Collins, explores the reality of living in spite of a head injury and a spinal cord injury. It considers the complexities related to being a survivor, a husband, a father, and an emerging person who is challenging the future and transcending the past.

Personal Statement

FOR BETTER OR FOR WORSE
by David Collins

Growing up in a family, as the youngest of three boys, competition and survival were somewhat innate qualities. Athletics followed and play an important part of my life. During high school, my time was spent practicing for the upcoming game and "getting by" in the classroom to maintain eligibility. In college, my priorities changed and academics was a goal I pursued to stay out of the draft more than anything else. At 23, Valerie, the lady I met in college, and I walked down the church aisle and professed our love to those in attendance. Nine months and three days later, we welcomed an arrival to our union. As a coach and teacher, my skills were enhanced at classes or clinics; parenting I hoped would be a natural talent. As Kerry started to grow and reach her second birthday, we were good pals. If she misbehaved, this ex-coach would make her sit on her plastic chair and not get up. Probably a theory I had read about from one of my coaching journals. As Kerry grew, so did Valerie. She was expecting our second child in April. After some thinking, I chose to give up the coaching and get into real estate sales and H & R Block tax work. Now with a family it was important to look to the future and be prepared! I would make my mark and my family would enjoy the benefits. My planning was poor in implementing this action. After I played my "last" Christmas basketball game with fellow coaches, we convened at the local pub to review the game. After drinking beer and eating breakfast, I got in my car to drive home. Halfway home, I fell asleep and struck a utility pole while sitting atop my seat belt. My life was instantaneously altered. As my pregnant wife entered the hospital emergency room at 4:00 a.m., the neurosurgeon blasted her about my alcohol content and prognosis being, if I survived, needing constant attention. The accident was December 27th. My first recollection was in March, watching the state high school basketball tournament. I called my wife by her maiden name, asked if we had any children, and displayed not only confusion, but an indifference as well. At one point, I was convinced they had wheeled my bed up a floor to the OB section, and in my mind I vividly remembered delivering a baby. My days were spent going down to therapy and returning to bed and watching television. A young man started visiting me in my room and sharing his story with me. Turns out this fellow named Dave had fallen out of a tree seven years prior, when he was 16 years old, and broken his back. He was very muscular as he wheeled around the halls and explained things to me like driving a car with hand controls, keeping bowel and bladder control, and sexual activities with his dates. Dave got me out of my room and wheeling outside; he explained his life in graduate school to me and it was appealing. In time I chose to attend graduate school at the University of Illinois, renowned for its accessible campus and wheelchair sports programs. After six months in the hospital and plans being made for discharge, I was allowed to go home for weekend passes. My expectations were upon returning home that everything from my relations with my daughter to my relation to my wife would be as they were before. My foremost thought was to resume sexual activity with Valerie and provide for both our needs. At 27, I had serious doubts about being a person or a man, and felt the only way to prove my virility was in the bedroom. Valerie was very patient and empathic to my needs. My hygiene was terrible, a trache was in place on my throat, my bladder and bowel needed to be emptied prior to commencing intimacy, and there was always the chance of having an accident. To this day, I will always be indebted to her for allowing me to believe "I was a man." Teasingly, she is told she gave Oscar winning performances–when I needed them.

When I made it home for keeps, and re-entered the family unit, it had become blatantly apparent that Kerry, our precocious three-year-old, had taken my place. She had to be moved out of the king-size bed, back to her room. My adjustment to returning home, I had told Valerie, would be unnoticeable–or so I thought. My first morning home, I had forgotten to put my clothes next to my bed on the wheelchair (dressing is done prone on the bed). After 15 minutes of yelling for Valerie, finally I got, "Yeah what," to which I requested she get my pants for me that were on the floor. "I'm changing the baby and can't get back to you for 45 minutes." I was livid; "bullshit," I mumbled as I got in my chair, retrieved my trousers, and, getting back in bed, got dressed. Upon coming out to the kitchen and observing Valerie drinking coffee and reading a magazine, I let loose. What in the hell is going on, and after five minutes of ranting, I stormed off. Valerie and I put on several workshops/seminars on coping, etc., to healthcare professionals and families. We refer to this as the "Pants Story," and the lesson we convey is never again did I ever forget my pants. I'm sure it was hard for Valerie to hear my pleas and not give in, but the lesson we learned is it is a disservice to perform a task for an individual without his/her attempting the feat.

As time progressed, I entered graduate school and, due to the insight of the DVR Counselor, who suggested that only two courses be taken to start out, I succeeded. As I wheeled across the street on a campus of 45,000 students, my name was yelled out and I stopped. A fellow came up and asked, "Didn't you play basketball for Brother Rice in Chicago?" "Yeah," I said, and as we continued our discussion, he was recognized as a wide receiver for a rival high school in Chicago. He went on to tell me he was pursuing his Ph.D. in Therapeutic Recreation/ Administration. In the next sentence, he asked if I would be interested in going out for the track team. My first thoughts were, 'hope he is not in a hurry to get his Ph.D. after that question.' The look of bewilderment on my face led him to explain therapeutic recreation and how the University of Illinois had a wheelchair track, basketball, football, and a variety of other sports for those who are physically challenged. Practices were to start in the armory in two weeks. At my first practice, I was amazed to see the number of participants and their varying levels of function. I started to bring my daughter to practices and all of us seemed to enjoy ourselves. At various meets, my girls would get with me when ribbons were awarded and have their pictures taken–each of us were proud. The practices and the meets turned into family outings for us all. Valerie coordinated things well by loading up the car with kids, a wheelchair, and me. I could sense becoming less competitive with the girls.

As they became older, they became interested in playing sports. As a former coach, I had to use verbal restraint as I cheered on from the sidelines at their t-ball games. One parent asked me if I would assist him in coaching the girls' basketball team that both our daughters were members of. Reluctantly I agreed, but again my daughters were proud of their dad sitting on the courtside bench. We truly began to communicate better and spoke about events that happened in the practices or games.

I followed both girls as they progressed through the years. When they were younger, they didn't know that fathers on wheelchairs weren't cool. As they grew older, their parents knew less than they did, but I could tell that had nothing to do with my being in a wheelchair–just a normal attitude/reaction to parents. One time, as I pulled into a mall, Kerry asked, "Why do you park in wheelchair parking?" "Why not?" I replied. "You compete in 10K races and can wheel better than some of these older people can walk." I thought for a few minutes and felt somewhat flattered and responded, "Yeah, I suppose you're right." "It sounds like a special favor you're taking advantage of," she said. "I'll remember that in the future" was my nonverbal response.

It was August and both girls asked if I would drive them and their friends to an amusement park. Our group had about eight people waiting in a long line to ride the attraction. As we sweltered in 90+ temperature, a lady that took tickets came up to me and said, "Are you familiar with our wheelchair policy?" I said no, and she explained that any wheelchair patrons and their guests do not have to wait in line and may go to the front and stay on the ride for a second time if they chose. I looked at my oldest daughter and said, "I don't know. It kind of sounds like a special favor to me. What do you think?" "Oh no dad. This is okay this time." Later in the month, my wife offered to take the girls to the same amusement park to which they quickly responded, "Can dad come?"

In my family relationships with my spouse and my daughters, I have tried to live by showing that we all have choices–that sometimes because of our behavior we must accept the consequences. We all have special qualities and are unique. When we speak to others, communication is stressed as very important. Times are difficult for a lot of people and the key to my living is accepting and liking myself and taking one day at a time.

During graduate school, I went in to see the psychologist that worked at the rehabilitation center and inquired about what personal changes might I expect since traumatized and chaired. His response stayed with me and makes a lot of sense: "If you were an S.O.B. before using a wheelchair, the chances are, post trauma and using a chair, you will be an S.O.B. in a wheelchair. The point being, usually we don't plan bad things to happen to us: trauma, divorce, death, etc., but we still have the opportunity to change. Some are given a second chance, but that alone does not mean success. Like anyone else, we are all individuals who need to work on our relationships, within families as well as outside families. If we take one day at a time and keep a positive attitude, good things can result. In dealing with others, I clarify that my point is not to downplay or minimize trauma and its consequences–however, when one feels good about him/herself, regardless of the circumstances, they can share their routine feelings with others. Each of us has a choice–choice can never be taken away.

Allied health providers, all members in society, must recognize each individual as unique and possessive of skills others don't have. No two people are made alike–uniqueness in abilities is our gift to one another.

DISCUSSION QUESTIONS ON THE PERSONAL STATEMENT "FOR BETTER OR FOR WORSE"

1. What is lost/gained when a young athlete is faced with the changes subsequent to a disability? Are there any inherent or positive traits an athlete may possess to aid the process of rehabilitation?

2. How can long-term goals be a source of stress for a person whose life is altered by a head injury? How does this compare with the immediate stress related to hygiene, dressing, eating, etc.?

3. Is a single person with a head injury "better off" than a married person with young children? Is someone with a congenital disability "better off" than a person who experiences a mid-life trauma and must learn to adapt at age 50 to the demands related to activities of daily living?

4. How does the problematic relationship between alcohol and athletics manifest itself? Are roles of self-esteem and peer pressure relevant and contributory?

5. Was the response of the neurosurgeon helpful to David's wife?

6. How would you respond if your spouse did not remember who you were and whether or not you had children?

7. How can exposure to role models be a positive or stressful experience? (e.g., having David meet with an active person who has mastered his disability).

8. How can the need for intimacy become a major priority for a person returning home from the hospital? How did Valerie facilitate the adjustment?

9. How could the re-entry into the family have been facilitated by a creative discharge planning process?

10. How would your spouse respond if he or she had to choose between your needs and those of a child?

11. Why were sports a critical element in David's adjustment to his family?

12. What are the issues for children in adjusting to a parent with a head injury? How is the age of a child a mitigating factor in the adjustment process?

13. What does David mean when he states, "Each of us had a choice."?

14. What would your challenges be if you were in David's situation?

15. How can a person or a family be proactive in the adjustment to a head injury?

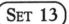

SET 13

WHY US?

Perspective: Most families live life hoping and expecting they will avoid the traumas and tragedies that are part of the life experience. No one can find fault with this perspective and hopefully most families will avoid the overwhelming traumas, tragedies, and losses that do occur. However, when a trauma does occur it becomes an integral part of the family's life experience. In these situations, most families tend to focus their resources and make the necessary accommodations and often reach a level of life functioning that is balanced and manageable. The vulnerability of most families in this situation is that they believe that nothing could be worse. Unfortunately, one trauma or one head injury does not make a person immune or insulated from additional loss and grief.

Loss, grief, and bereavement are part of the life and living process. Unfortunately, the losses and the subsequent grief are often sad, painful and distressing.

With a head injury, the losses my be major, minor, or somewhere in between. Often the loss associated with a head injury is magnified by prior losses and the unresolved pain associated with the loss experience.

Exploration:
1. What was the most important thing you have lost in your life?
2. Who was the most important person you have lost?
3. What have you done or not done to help you resolve the loss and minimize the pain?
4. How has or how would a head injury experience intensity prior losses?
5. What advice, help or insights could you give a family member who cannot get beyond focusing upon what they have lost as a result of a head injury?
6. How would you and your family feel and act if you sustained a traumatic brain injury, recovered and were diagnosed with multiple sclerosis?
7. How would you feel if you had a head injury and your spouse decided to place you in a nursing home so that better care could be given to your child who had a chronic illness?
8. Identify and discuss how relationships with others have changed during your life span.
9. Were any of these changes a result of unresolved issues between family members related to illness, disability or death?
10. What message has your family given to you regarding why people are injured?
11. What would be the first thing your family would say to you if you were head injured because you were driving while under the influence of alcohol?
12. How would your spouse respond if you refused to buy a bicycle helmet for your child and as a result the child sustained a head injury?

REFERENCES

Anthony, W., & Carkhuff, R. (1976). *The art of health care*. Amherst: MA. Human Resource Development Press.

Bowlby, J. (1961). Process of mourning. *International Journal of Psychoanalysis, 42*, 315-382.

Bowlby, J. (1973). *Attachment and loss*. New York: Basic Books.

Brown, J. C. (1990). Loss and grief: An overview and guided imagery intervention model. *Journal of Mental Health Counseling, 12*(4), 434-445.

Brown, T. J., & Stoudemine, A. G. (1983). Normal and pathological grief. *Journal of the American Medical Association, 250*, 378-382.

Bugen, L. A. (1977). Human grief: A model for prediction and intervention. *American Journal of Orthopsychiatry, 47*, 196-206.

Kane, B. (1990). Grief and the adaptation to loss. *Rehabilitation Education, 4*, 213-224.

Kubler-Ross, E. (1969). *On death and dying*. New York: MacMillan.

Matz, M. (1978). Helping families cope with grief. In S. Eisenberg & L. Patterson (Eds.), *Helping clients with special concerns* (pp.218-238). Chicago: Rand McNally College Publishing Co.

McKinlay, W., & Hickox, A. (1988). How can families help in the rehabilitation of the head injured? *Journal of Head Trauma Rehabilitation, 3*(4), 64-72.

9

GROUP COUNSELING: A RESOURCE FOR PERSONS AND FAMILIES CHALLENGED BY A HEAD INJURY

9

GROUP COUNSELING: A RESOURCE FOR PERSONS AND FAMILIES CHALLENGED BY A HEAD INJURY

PERSPECTIVE

Like many other illnesses and disabilities, head injury creates new roles, expectations, challenges, and demands for the person with the injury, as well as for their family.

Consequently, health care professionals need to understand the encompassing nature of disability when developing intervention, treatment and rehabilitation strategies. Group counseling has been presented as a resource that can respond to the complex and changing needs of persons and families challenged by the illness or disability experience (Baider, 1989; D'Afflitti & Weitz, 1974; Dispenza & Nigro, 1989; Hedge & Glover, 1990; Hoge & McLoughlin, 1991; Holmes, Karst & Goodwin, 1990; Huberty, 1980; Johnson & Stark, 1980; Lonergan, 1982; Mack & Berman, 1988; McKelvey & Borgersen, 1990; Ross, 1979, Roy, Flynn, & Atcherson, 1982; Seligman, 1990; Sheahen, 1984; Steinglass, Gonzalez, Dosovitz, & Reiss, 1982; Szivos & Griffiths, 1990; Taylor, Falke, Shoptaw, & Lichtman, 1986; Videka-Sherman & Lieberman, 1985; Walwork, 1984; Wasserman & Danforth, 1988; Wellisch, Mosher, & Van Scoy, 1978; Westin & Reiss, 1979; Yalom, 1985; Zimpfer, 1989).

GROUP COUNSELING AND HEAD INJURY

When group counseling is applied to head injury treatment and rehabilitation, it can become a counter-force to helplessness, isolation, and desperation because it brings people together to share their individual concerns as well as to develop their common resources.

A major contribution of group counseling, when applied to head injury treatment and rehabilitation, is that it provides an opportunity for people to explore the dimensions of their experiences and needs while developing skills to maximize their resources through a peer-oriented and goal-oriented support system. Group counseling can: a) help put head injury into perspective, b) facilitate the development of resources, c) support both the client and the family during the process of treatment and rehabilitation, d) expose individuals and families to role models, and e) teach the necessary skills to effectively respond to past, present, and future concerns. As a result of the demonstrated value of groups, group counseling with families and individuals experiencing a head injury is becoming an integral part of treatment and rehabilitation (Abramsom, 1975; Campbell, 1988; Frye, 1982; Hegeman, 1988; Jarman & Stone, 1989; Mauss-Clum & Ryan, 1981; Quinn, Ford, & Mazzawy, 1981; Rosenthal, 1987; Rosenthal & Young, 1988; Valancy, 1981; Williams, 1987; Zeigler, 1989).

CRITICAL ISSUES RELATED TO GROUP COUNSELING WITH FAMILIES EXPERIENCING A HEAD INJURY

There are many consequences of a head injury experience that can intensify the trauma and deplete personal and family resources. Some of these consequences are:

1. Marital relationships can begin to deteriorate, and spouses may see separation, resignation or divorce as the only way to save and remove themselves from a situation they cannot handle. (Lezak, 1978; McLaughlin & Schaffer, 1985; Zeigler, 1989)

2. Siblings may act out as a result of the changes in the family and experience resentment, jealousy, and parental pressure (Orsillo, S. M., McCaffrey, R. J., & Fisher, J. M., 1993; Waaland & Kreutzer, 1988).

3. Substance abuse of a family member may develop as a means to cope with the stress and losses associated with a head injury. (Waaland & Kreutzer, 1988)

4. Work performance of the injured family member may deteriorate and result in loss of job (Jacobs, 1988).

5. Individual family members, as well as the total family can neglect themselves both physically and emotionally by not tending to individual or mutual needs (Hegeman, 1988).

6. Financial pressures can be seen as a cause of disharmony when, in fact, they may be symptomatic of underlying global stress that is more difficult to concretize. DeJong, Batavia, and Williams (1990) stated:

    The costs of medical care, personal care, supervision, residential care and respite care for a person with a head injury can quickly exhaust the financial capacities of even the most prosperous families. (p.13)

    While focusing on financial costs the authors make reference to the emotional costs and the similar depletion of emotional resources that can also occur.

7. Traditional support systems, such as friends and relatives, may remove themselves from supporting roles because of their inability to respond to the emotional demands made upon them. (Armstrong, 1991; Jarman & Stone, 1989; Lezak, 1978). The challenge of group counseling is to address these concerns, manage a complex reality and provide families with a structure and process to control their reactions while developing their resources. One of the most powerful insights that can take place in a group is the awareness that group members are not alone and that there are others who can help them to process what has happened as well as help prepare them for what will occur. The importance of groups is discussed by Rosenthal (1987) when he states:

    ...groups offer opportunities to share common experiences, problems, and solutions; vent frustration and anger; and provide emotional support. Often, family members obtain specific information about community-based resources that can aid their relative. (p.56)

    In such groups, members are able to participate in an unfolding process that gradually prepares them to face and adjust to their own individual loss. In a sense, it is an opportunity to see similar people faced with similar loss, who still can cope while maintaining control over their lives.

Group Leadership and Head Injury

Leaders of groups that deal with families involved in the head injury experience must be highly skilled. They must have a broad perspective on head injury, possess group leadership skills, be personally integrated, and have the ability to cognitively and experientially appreciate the impact of head injury, loss and trauma on the person and on the family.

The following is a list of some of the characteristics and skills which can be helpful to the role and functioning of a group leader:

1. Humaneness–an appreciation of the plight, struggle, needs, fears and hopes of families, which manifests itself in a caring kind, empathetic, and helpful manner.
2. Compassion–the ability to feel in a constructive way.
3. Resiliency–the ability to continue with the tasks of one's role in spite of personal emotional drain, which often accompanies a repetition of "failure" experiences or personal loss which may be consequent to head injury treatment and rehabilitation.
4. Intervention skills–ability to design and implement programs and responses that are timely, creative, visionary and relevant to the changing needs of the person and family.
5. Medical knowledge–the ability to comprehend complexities of a head injury and its impact on the patient, the family, and the group process.
6. Communication skills–the ability to relate to person, family, significant others and members of the interdisciplinary health care team.
7. Ability to differentiate between individual and family problems.
8. Awareness of the synergistic effect head injury and other situations can have on the group process, the individual, and the family system.
9. Ability to orchestrate group process with complex themes.
10. Awareness of the independent and conjoint functioning of family subsystems.
11. Ability to be proactive rather than reactive.
12. Ability to work with a co-leader, which is helpful with large groups and provides a feedback and support system for leaders.
13. Ability to resolve personal prejudices as they relate to the potential and liabilities of clients and their family members.
14. Cognitive and experiential awareness of head injury and its consequences. Group leaders should have experienced a training format which focuses on what head injury means to the person and the family, and what it would mean for them as well as their families. The ideal is to have a co-leader who personally has experienced the reality of a head injury within their family. However, personal experience alone is not adequate just as a professional degree does not always equate with effectiveness.
15. Comprehensive understanding of a model that is relevant, applicable, and useful to families challenged by head injury who are engaged in a life-long journey and

not just a destination. While group leaders must have at their command a variety of skills, resources and perspectives, a group model can be more responsive to complex needs if it is comprehensive, proactive and multidimensional.

The need for a multidimensional model is reflected in a statement by Holmes, Karst, and Goodwin (1990), in a discussion of the role and contribution of mutual help groups to the rehabilitation process. They state:

> Mutual help groups typically provide members with a variety of services aimed at helping them achieve specific goals. Specific services can include transportation, employment information and education, disability education and service information, family and individual social support, daily living skills training, peer counseling, community exploration, personal advice, planned entertainment, self-advocacy training, help with problem resolution and financial information (p.21).

MULTIDIMENSIONAL GROUP MODEL

A viable group counseling model must go beyond a token response to the needs of families and individuals living with a head injury. This can occur when a group counseling program addresses issues encountered and anticipated during the treatment, rehabilitation and life and living process.

A multidimensional group counseling model for persons with head injury and their families should be designed to be comprehensive and proactive rather than limited and reactive. A comprehensive proactive group model is one that:

1. Is available throughout the head injury experience.
2. Has the potential to be adapted to a variety of settings (e.g., community, home, hospital, independent living, or rehabilitation facility).
3. Is flexible to meet the evolving and changing needs of the person and the family.
4. Can be fully integrated into a rehabilitation program.
5. Is capable of transcending the hospital environment and meeting the demands faced in the community.
6. Has didactic components to teach the skills needed to respond to a range of medical and nonmedical problems related to the head injury experience.
7. Can respond to the life losses that may have an important role in adjustment to the head injury experience.
8. Is capable of anticipating problems rather than only reacting to them.

With a multidimensional group model, the needs of the families can be better met by providing a system of alternatives as well as a system of supplementary groups. The following is a list of potential subgroups and their focus.

- **Family Group**—The family group is the central, core group, focusing on family issues. It is from this group that the other groups evolve.
- **Peer Group**—Focuses on needs of the person in a group setting with peers.
- **Female Group**—Addresses role issues that are relative to female issues and concerns.
- **Male Group**—Addresses role issues that are relative to male issues and concerns.
- **Children's/Sibling Group**—Opportunity for children to share feelings and learn how to respond to their unique situations (e.g., the injury of a parent or the stress related to a sibling being in a coma management program).
- **Spouse/Marital Group**—Concerned with nurturing and maintaining a realistic marital relationship while coping with head injury. The importance of this group is stated by Zeigler (1989):

  Spouses of head injury survivors face particular problems which are often not addressed in head injury family support groups. These issues can be effectively dealt with in mutual support groups. Since the number of spouses affected by brain injury is less than the number of parents who are affected, the availability of spouse support groups is limited. These groups do seem to be emerging in various parts of the country utilizing a variety of formats. (p.37)

- **Care Giver and Significant Others Group**—An opportunity to involve those persons who are a part of the families' or clients' interactional system (Armstrong, 1991).
- **Didactic Group**—Provides information and teaches relevant skills related to living in spite of a head injury.
- **Theme Group**—Permits the addressing of various issues related to the head injury experience.
- **Medical Staff Group**—Opportunity for health and human care workers to discuss issues relative to their individual functioning and to provide a professional support system.
- **Vocational Rehabilitation Group**—Addressing issues related to employment and careers.
- **Life and Living Group**—Focusing on the process of developing a quality of life and living in spite of a head injury.

While these are some examples of potential subgroups, Hill and Carper (1985), in an article focusing on group therapeutic approaches with persons with a head injury, identified a variety of other groups offered in a rehabilitation facility. The groups offered included: a) speech-language groups, b) education groups, c) recreation groups, d) occupational therapy groups, e) nutrition groups, f) psychotherapy groups, and g) physical therapy groups. While recognizing that there are advantages in group work with persons who have had a head injury, Hill and Carper state: "The use of groups for cognitive rehabilitation can offer motivation, new learnings and socialization for patients." (Hill & Carper, 1985, p.26). However, it is important to recognize that group counseling is not a "magic" solution to all the problems, concerns and needs of this population. For some individuals, group settings may not be appropriate due to the nature and complexity of their limitations. In such situations, the criteria for group intervention must be whether or not a group will be an additive to a person's life and living experience.

CONCLUSION

Group counseling is a valuable resource in working with the family and person challenged by a head injury experience. A comprehensive, relevant and available group counseling program is a means to:

1. Expose families coping with head injury to role models who were able or are trying to meet the life and living challenges posed by the head injury of a family member.

2. Provide a support system that will respond to the evolving and changing long-term needs throughout the head injury experience rather than be limited to the concerns associated with acute care.

3. Create a structure within which family members can respond to their individual as well as collective needs and receive support, understanding and encouragement from persons in similar as well as dissimilar situations.

4. Introduce family members to other resources based upon the knowledge and expertise of other group members. This avoids the unnecessary strain and stress of individual families having to struggle for information that is already available. A valuable resource for such information is The National Head Injury Foundation and other national, regional and local agencies. (Appendix A and B)

5. Teach families how to cope by developing a proactive rather than a reactive response to problems that are common to life and living after a head injury.

6. Provide a structure for the introduction of medical knowledge that is relevant and helpful to group members.

7. Establish a consumer point of view in a professional world and facilitate dialogue with health care and rehabilitation workers.

8. Create a level of accountability for all who are involved in the treatment of persons with head injury. A collective of families and significant others is often more aware of what should be happening compared with an individual family in a state of crisis.

9. Diffuse problems before they become overwhelming to the family or its individual members. This can be accomplished by exposing families to the problems and solutions employed by other group members.

10. Enable families to share the common burden of head injury rather than be fragmented by the desperation that is often a by-product of isolation.

11. Personalize the treatment process by processing information in a caring, structured manner rather than in an impersonal, random, unstructured manner.

12. Develop the group as a referral source that can result in professional, personal and social contacts, which are essential in coping with head injury over an extended period of time.

13. Understand that the existence of a group counseling program does not mean that all problems related to head injury can be solved, but it can mean that critical elements in the head injury experience will have a better chance of being attended to.

Group counseling with families and individuals challenged by a head injury is a major resource in personalizing the health care system and providing a vehicle for support, skills, mutuality, sensitivity, honesty, caring, concern, and consistency that can facilitate the adjustment to living with the effects and realities associated with a head injury.

The major contribution of group counseling is that people can share their pain and hope, while realizing that they are not alone. The following personal statement, "Better Than Being Alone," focuses on the need for significant others.

Personal Statement

BETTER THAN BEING ALONE
(A Husband's Perspective)

The worst part of having my wife become head injured was the feeling that nothing like this has happened to anyone before. Here I was, 41 years old, happy, and content. I was healthy, my 39-year-old wife was successful in her business, and our children were all doing very well. Nowhere in my background had I ever been exposed to a major illness or even considered it happening to me or my family.

On a tranquil fall evening in 1987, my wife sustained a severe head injury when she was struck by a speeding car while walking our dog. Fortunately, a passing motorist saw the dog standing next to my wife who was lying on the roadside, and immediately called for help. I was notified by the police and did not realize the seriousness of the situation until I was confronted with the reality of the emergency room. At this point, I realized that I was not prepared for the seriousness of the injury nor did I realize what was in store for my wife, children, or family. The next five months were a blur. I was terrified, confused, and uncertain as to what to expect. My family and friends were supportive, but not helpful. They were equally in shock and were just as overwhelmed as I.

When my wife began rehabilitation, I was delighted that she had survived, but I was not sure I could cope with how she had changed or deal with an uncertain future. Fortunately, I met a woman whose husband had been injured and who was a member of a support group. After sharing our stories, she suggested that I join the group (which I did, but with very mixed feelings).

First of all, I found it very difficult to talk to strangers about personal things. Secondly, I was not sure what to expect or whether or not it would be helpful. At the first meeting, I was surprised to see 11 other people who all had family members with a head injury. While some had children, siblings, spouses, or relatives, all shared the common bond of being in a very difficult place and not wanting to have to deal with the situation.

During the next several group meetings, I mostly listened, observed, and talked about superficial things. I also began to read the literature that was available and began to realize that there was a lot more to this head injury stuff than I realized or wanted to hear. As painful as it was, it was helpful to begin to realize what I was up against.

In time, I became more comfortable with the group and began to realize that some people were doing better than others. I also heard people talk about wanting to run away, get divorced, or make a bad situation better. This range of feelings enabled me to share my feelings and also to get support and understanding from a group of people who shared my common fears, as well as dreams. Also, it was helpful to realize that I personally had choices. There were things I could do or not do. This helped me realize that I did not have to be a victim.

My most difficult challenge was to realize that my wife may not get better and that she could even get worse. This was very scary for me and it was helpful to see other group members who were able to keep their focus on the big picture and consider their own needs and those of their family. While the group did not directly change my situation, it gave me hope, support, and perspective. It also helped me to establish a network of people who help me gain my bearings, help my children, and make me realize that I needed a lot of help from my friends and that it was a lot better than being alone.

DISCUSSION QUESTIONS ON THE PERSONAL STATEMENT

1. What are the advantages and disadvantages of not experiencing serious illness and trauma?

2. Discuss how the circumstances related to the onset of a head injury can help or impede familiar and personal adjustment (e.g., in this case, the fact that the hit and run driver was never caught).

3. In this situation, when should the family have access to a family support group?

4. Do you think that family groups should be limited to only individuals who have a spouse or child who is head injured? What are advantages and disadvantages of having mixed groups?

5. Is it helpful to have group members be exposed to situations that are much worse or much better than their own?

6. How long do you think a support group should be available to people with head injuries, as well as their families?

(SET 14)

COMMON PAIN, MUTUAL SUPPORT

Perspective: A harsh reality of illness and disability is that individuals and families are often abandoned, isolated and left on their own. Group counseling can provide a helpful alternative for families challenged by a head injury by providing structure, support and resources at a time of ongoing crisis. When thinking about group counseling and self-help alternatives, it is important to recognize some families are not accustomed to sharing feelings with strangers and may resist the group counseling experience. In such cases, gradual exposure to group members may create the needed bridges to help families find a common ground and become receptive to a group experience.

Exploration:
1. List five ways group counseling could help you and your family adjust to living with the effects of a head injury.
2. If you had a head injury, would you voluntarily enter a group? Why or why not?
3. What would be the most difficult aspect of group counseling for you as a group member?
4. What would be the most difficult aspect for you as a group leader?
5. Are there certain people with illnesses or disabilities you would not want to associate with?
6. List the characteristics of group members that make you uncomfortable.
7. If you could choose a group leader to lead a group for persons and families experiencing a head injury, what would be ten characteristics you would like this person to have?
8. What are the characteristics of a group leader that would put you off?
9. Do you feel that you are fully functioning in your own life so that you are a role model for others?
10. Would this change if you became head injured?
11. What is the ideal size of a group for persons with a head injury?
12. Identify the most upsetting situation that could occur for you as a group member and as a leader.
13. How long should each group session be?
14. Should people with a disability and people without a disability be in the same group? Why or why not?
15. Should persons with a head injury be in a group with individuals who are living with AIDS, spinal cord injury or mental retardation?
16. Do you prefer a group model that stresses structure or feelings?
17. What are the characteristics of a group experience that are important for persons and families living with a head injury?
18. How long should a group experience last? Weeks? Months? Years?
19. What are the advantages and disadvantages of having families coping with illness such as stroke, cancer, with AIDS, etc. participate in the same group as families impacted by a head injury?
20. Are there issues that should not be discussed in a group experience?
21. Should a family ever be excluded from a self-help or family group program?

22. Should groups be led by family members?
23. What are the advantages and disadvantages of "professionally" led groups? Groups led by survivors?
24. From your perspective, what is the primary goal of group counseling?
25. Should the person with a head injury always be part of the family group?
26. What are the disadvantages and limitations of a group counseling program for families living the head injury experience?
27. At what point during treatment and rehabilitation should family members join a group?
28. Identify and discuss some reasonable expectations that family members may have of the group process.

References

Abramson, M. (1975). Group treatment of families of brain-injured patients. *Social Casework, 56,* 235-241.

Armstrong, C. (1991, June). Emotional changes following brain injury: Psychological and neurological components of depression, denial and anxiety. *Journal of Rehabilitation,* pp. 15-22.

Baider, L. (1989). Group therapy with adolescent cancer patients. *Journal of Adolescent Health Care, 10*(1), 35-38.

Campbell, C. H. (1988). Needs of relatives and helpfulness of support groups in severe head injury. *Rehabilitation Nursing, 13,* 6, 320-325.

D'Afflitti, J. D., & Weitz, G. W. (1974). Rehabilitating the stroke patient through patient-family groups. *International Journal of Group Psychotherapy, 25,* 327-332.

DeJong, G., Batavia, A. I., & Williams, J. M. (1990). Who is responsible for the lifelong well being of a person with a head injury? *Journal of Head Trauma and Rehabilitation, 5*(1), 9-22.

Dispenza, D. A., & Nigro, A. G. (1989). Life skills for the mentally ill: A program description. *Journal of Applied Rehabilitation Counseling, 20*(1), 47-49.

Frye, B. A. (1982). Brain injury and family education needs. *Rehabilitation Nursing, 7,* 27-28.

Hedge, B., & Glover, L. F. (1990). Group intervention with HIV seropositive patients and their partners. *AIDS Care, 2*(2), 147-154.

Hegeman, K. M. (1988). A care plan for the family of a brain trauma client. *Rehabilitation Nursing, 13,* 5, 254-259.

Hill, J., & Carper, M. (1985, Jan./Feb.). Greenery: Group therapeutic approaches with the head injured. *Cognitive Rehabilitation,* pp. 18-29.

Hoge, M. A., & McLoughlin, K. A. (1991). Group psychotherapy in acute treatment settings: Theory and technique. *Hospital and Community Psychiatry, 42*(2), 153-158.

Holmes, G. E., Karst, R., & Goodwin, L. R. (1990, Autumn). Mutual help groups and the rehabilitation process. *American Rehabilitation,* pp. 19-22.

Huberty, D. (1980). Adapting to illness through family groups. In P. W. Power & A. E. Dell Orto (Eds.), *Role of the family in the rehabilitation of the physically disabled.* Baltimore: University Park Press.

Jacobs, H. E. (1988). The Los Angeles head injury survey: Procedures and initial findings. *Archives of Physical Medicine and Rehabilitation, 69,* 425-431.

Jarman, D. J., & Stone, J. A. (1989, May/June). Brain injury: Issues and benefits arising within a family support group. *Cognitive Rehabilitation,* pp. 30-33.

Johnson, E. M., & Stark, D. E. (1980). A group program for cancer patients and their family members in an acute care teaching hospital. *Social Work in Health Care, 5,* 335-349.

Lezak, M. (1978). Living with the characterologically altered brain injured patient. *Journal of Clinical Psychiatry, 39,* 592-598.

Lonergan, E. C. (1982). *Group intervention: How to begin and maintain groups in medical and psychiatric settings.* New York: Jason Aronson.

Mack, S. A., & Berman, L. C. (1988). A group for parents of children with fatal genetic illness. *American Journal of Orthopsychiatry, 58,* 397-404.

Mauss-Clum, N., & Ryan, M. (1981). Brain injury and the family. *Journal of Neurosurgical Nursing, 13,* 165-169.

McKelvey, J., & Borgersen, M. (1990). Family development and the use of diabetes groups: Experience with a model approach. *Patient Education and Counseling, 16*(1), 61-67.

McLaughlin, A. M., & Schaffer, V. (1985). Rehabilitate or remold? Family involvement in head trauma recovery. *Cognitive Rehabilitation, 3*(1), 14-17.

Orsillo, S. M., McCaffrey, R. J., & Fisher, J. M. (1993). Siblings of head-injured individuals: A population at risk. *Journal of Head Trauma Rehabilitation, 8*(1), 102-115.

Quinn, A., Ford, J., & Mazzawy, M. (1981). Families and feelings: A time for sharing. *Journal of Neurosurgical Nursing, 13,* 217-218.

Rosenthal, M. (1987). Traumatic head injury: Neurobehavioral consequences. In B. Caplan (Ed.) *Rehabilitation psychology desk reference.* Rockville, Aspen.

Rosenthal, M., & Young, T. (1988). Effective family intervention after traumatic brain injury: Theory and practice. *Journal of Head Trauma Rehabilitation, 3,* 4:42-50.

Ross, J. W. (1979). Coping with childhood cancer: Group intervention as an aid to parents in crisis. *Social Work in Health Care, 4*, 381-391.

Roy, C. A., Flynn, E., & Atcherson, E. (1982). Group sessions for home hemodialysis assistants. *Health and Social Work, 7*, 65-71.

Seligman, M. (1990). *Selecting effective treatments: A comprehensive, systematic guide to treating adult mental disorders.* San Francisco: Jossey-Bass.

Sheahen, M. C. (1984). Review of a support group for patients with AIDS. *Topics in Clinical Nursing, 6*, 38-44.

Steinglass, P., Gonzalez, S., Dosovitz, L., & Reiss, D. (1982). Discussion groups for chronic hemodialysis patients and their families. *General Hospital Psychiatry, 4*, 140-161.

Szivos, S. E., & Griffiths, E. (1990). Group processes involved in coming to terms with a mentally retarded identity. *Mental Retardation, 28*(6), 333-341.

Taylor, S. E., Falke, R. L., Shoptaw, S. J., & Lichtman, R.R. (1986). Social support, support groups, and the cancer patient. *Journal of Consulting and Clinical Psychology, 54*, 608-615.

Valancy, B. B. (1981). A staff-directed group for parents of neurologically impaired children. In P. Azarnoff & C. Hardgrove (Eds.), *The family in child health care* (pp. 189-198). New York: John Wiley.

Videka-Sherman, L., & Lieberman, M. (1985). The effects of self-help and psychotherapy intervention on child loss: The limits of recovery. *American Journal of Orthopsychiatry, 55*, 70-82.

Waaland, P. K., & Kreutzer, J. S. (1988). Family response to childhood traumatic brain injury. *Journal of Head Trauma Rehabilitation, 3*, (4), 51-63.

Walwork, E. (1984). Coping with the death of a newborn. In H. B. Roback (Ed.). *Helping parents and their families cope with medical problems.* San Francisco: Jossey-Bass.

Wasserman, H., & Danforth, H. E. (1988). *The human bond: Support groups and mutual aid.* New York: Springer.

Wellisch, D. K., Mosher, M. B., & Van Scoy, C. (1978). Management of family emotional stress: Family group therapy in a private oncology practice. *International Journal of Group Psychotherapy, 28*, 225-232.

Westin, M. T., & Reiss, D. (1979). The family role in rehabilitation. *Journal of Rehabilitation, 11*, 25-29.

Williams, J. (1987). *Head injury support groups.* Available from: National Head Injury Foundation, 1140 Connecticut Ave, N.W., Washington, D.C. 20036

Yalom, I. D. (1985). *The theory and practice of group psychotherapy* (3rd ed.). New York: Basic Books.

Zeigler, E. A. (1989, May-June). The importance of mutual support for spouses of head injury. Cognitive Rehabilitation, pp. 34-37.

Zimpfer, D. G. (1989). Groups for persons who have cancer. *The Journal for Specialists in Group Work, 14*(2), 98-104.

10

Respite Care: Its Critical Role In Coping With Head Injury

10

Respite Care: Its Critical Role In Coping With Head Injury

Perspective

Respite care is emerging as a vital and essential force which is often the only buffer between the family and the ravages of illness and disability (Botuck & Winsberg, 1991; Grant & McGrath, 1990; Lawton, Brody, Saperstein, & Grimes, 1989; Marks, 1987; Pearson & Deitrick, 1989; Rimmerman, 1989). However, a major problem in head injury treatment and rehabilitation is that may of the problems encountered by persons experiencing a head injury and their families are not directly caused by the head injury, but are often a result of the lack of respite care and other services that can be of great benefit to the family and the person with a head injury (Brown & McCormick, 1988; Campbell, 1988; Graff & Minnes, 1989; Ridley, 1989). This situation exists because health care and rehabilitation systems are designed to provide treatment based on the assumption that at some point in time the person, their family, or significant others will be able to develop the physical, financial and emotional resources necessary to contain the ravages of a head injury while maintaining a balanced existence. While fine in theory, the reality is that many people do not have a family or significant others who have unlimited emotional, financial and physical resources to respond to the evolving challenges of a head injury experience. As DeJong, Batavia, and Williams (1990) state:

> ...some head-injured persons have a supportive family, and some have no family; some are employable, and some are not; some have access to financial resources, and some have no resources. Therefore, the extent to which individuals must rely

> on family and society for support depends largely on their
> personal conditions and socioeconomic circumstances. (p.12)

The complex reality is that family members may be able to tolerate a life of self-denial for a few days or weeks, but no one can endure a regimen of emotional and social deprivation indefinitely without becoming physically ill, emotionally disturbed, or both (Oddy, Humphrey, & Uttley, 1978).

When discussing coping with head injury, therefore, it is imperative that the respite care needs of individuals as well as families be taken into consideration. Hegeman (1987) states that:

> The traumatically brain-injured client is not the only victim;
> the family and/or significant others suffer as well. Disruption in
> the lifestyle and the emotional strain on the family caused by the
> trauma result in complex, long-standing problems.

A similar point is made by Armstrong (1991) who states:

> Without the day to day experience of the patient's irresponsibil-
> ity, impulsivity, or other problems, or of the duties, other
> relatives can easily misperceive the caretaker as being too
> protective or restrictive, or too neglectful or uncaring. Examples
> of this are unending, and even those professionals who are most
> committed or most caring can make these mistakes. Only those
> who have experienced the daily vigilances of care and worry are
> likely to be fully grateful and emotionally supportive of the
> family's accomplishments in fostering the patient's improve-
> ments. (p.20)

DEFINITIONS

Considering the mission of respite care, it is important to evaluate how it is defined. Just as there is variability in the populations served, there are differences in the definitions of respite care.

In their outstanding book, *Respite Care*, Cohen and Warren (1985) provide the following statement:

> The definition of respite care as "the temporary care of a disabled
> individual for the purpose of providing relief to the primary
> caregiver" seems straightforward and noncontroversial. How-
> ever, in practice, there is considerable variation in the interpre-
> tation of the scope of services to be called respite care. One of
> these variations concerns the distinction between intermittent
> and ongoing services. Virtually all definitions of respite care
> include the idea of temporary services. (p.26)

The major problem with a time limited definition of respite care is that the needs, problems and concerns of both the patient and family may be fluctuating in nature and exist over a lifetime. This is especially true for the family of the person challenged by a head injury who often have long term needs and short term resources.

Another definition of respite care is presented by Pullo and Hahn (1979):

> The temporary and periodic provision of a range of services which prevent individual and family breakdown by relieving the caretaker of stress by giving continuous support and/or care to a dependent individual. These services are not meant to replace other specialized services provided to an individual in need of care. (p.1)

What is significant about this definition is that it conveys a sensitivity to the consequences of unchecked demands made on the family and recognizes that a family can be overwhelmed if consistent help is not provided. While the definitions of respite care focus upon the importance of providing relief for the family/caregiver, they also address the importance of available respite care programs.

Theoretically, the availability of such programs should reflect a match between need and resources. Unfortunately, the **need** most often is in excess of the resources which in turn may create stress and frustration on the part of those caregivers who are in need of, and more often, desperate for such services. The need for programs is stated by Waaland and Kreutzer (1988) who point out that traditional respite care programs "are frequently unavailable to the child with a traumatic brain injury."

NEED

In order to better understand the family's need for respite care, it is important to recognize the developmental process which is associated with a head injury. Since a head injury does not impact everyone at the same point in the life span, it is imperative that respite care programs have the potential to respond to an evolving and changing need system. While the nature of the head injury plays a major role in the determination of need, consideration must also be given to the complexities surrounding the emerging interaction between the family and the patient as well as their changing needs and roles.

First, there are the needs of the family member directly challenged by head injury. These needs vary according to the intensity of physical and emotional aspects of the disability as well as the age of the person, their role in the family and their potential to maintain a degree of self dignity based on what was as well as what is and what will be. Secondly, the needs of the family vary according to its structure, resources, traditions, developmental stage and its ability to access support and accept the demands of the head injury experience.

These individual and familial needs, however, do not exist in isolation from the community, society, or the health care system. As DeJong, Batavia and Williams (1990) state:

> If the responsibility for persons with head injury were truly a shared obligation, the perceived burden of everyday caring by families would lighten substantially while the increased burden on the community and society would remain manageable. (p.21)

Even if the basic roles and functions of these systems are distinct from those of the family, these systems should be complimentary to the respite care goals and familial needs and not adversarial to them. Unfortunately, most health care and political systems are burdened with primary concern in the areas of policy and finances while consumers of respite care and their families are often concerned about more basic concerns such as emotional survival and quality of life. This point is made by Durgin (1989) when he states:

> It is critical that family members be aware of their limitations and not feel pressured to take on too much responsibility. Typically, there are a large number of professionals involved in rehabilitation because it is too extreme a challenge for one to "shoulder it all." Families should be sure to say "no" when they cannot take on more and should also let it be known when they would like to be more involved. (p.22)

For families with a characterologically altered head injured member, the issue of respite care is cast in the shadow of an often harsh, frustrating and demanding reality. In this situation, there is an intensification of the responsibilities and consequences of care. Rosenthal and Young (1988) state:

> The chronic nature of the brain injury will prohibit the family from returning to the kind of stability that was characteristic of its functioning prior to the injury. As the family cares for the characterologically altered family member, each person's own emotional and developmental needs become secondary to the management of the brain-injured person within the family. (p.45)

This is further complicated because families may be put in a position of having to choose between their emotional and physical stability or the care of a member having a head injury. For example, some family members may want to keep the person at home while others want to place the person in a long term care facility. In such cases, respite care options often can be the difference between a family being able to make life care choices from a position of strength rather than default. The complexity of these choices is addressed by Jarman and Stone (1989) when they state:

> Some parents may find they simply cannot provide the care their
> loved one needs, no matter how hard they try. At this point they
> agonize over the right decision, and are forced to acknowledge
> that they cannot make it "all better" for their injured child.
> Considering placement and alternative living options becomes
> a very difficult decision-making process for these parents. (p.32)

GENDER ISSUES AND ROLE FLEXIBILITY

The need for respite care does not differentiate between the
gender of the patient or that of the primary care given. Traditionally,
the woman has been designated by choice, tradition, or default, to
be the provider of "nurturance and care" (Zeigler, 1989).

While there have been gains in the emergence of new roles for
both women and men, there is still concern expressed regarding the
ability of people to make the role modifications necessary to respond
to the specific needs of a loved one or the complex demands of the
respite care process (Stroker, 1983). Therefore, role flexibility and
adaptability is key to a person being able to alter their personal goals,
aspirations and needs for the benefit of the total family system. While
difficult in the best of circumstances, this is almost impossible when
elements of dysfunction foster role rigidity, interpersonal stress, and
familial chaos. Consequently, there are few families that can make
the transition from wellness to state of loss and respond constructively if their prior interactions have been dysfunctional. Those
families that work together, who care about each other and have
functional role models are often the ones who can make the
adjustments that are helpful rather than helpless. As Waaland and
Kreutzer (1988) state:

> It is thus important that clinicians help families to mobilize
> effective resources and avoid mutual blaming or unhealthy
> family realignments that preclude marital health or clear
> generational boundaries. (p.57)

While family history, personal experiences, and role models can
be important factors in creating the perspective needed to meet the
demands of a head injury experience, the outcomes are not always
ideal. For example, if the caring for a head injured family member has
created a significant amount of family stress, the family may decide
that they will never place themselves in a similar situation. However
some families may be able to recognize why the situation was so
stressful and make changes which can reduce stress and make the
future situations more bearable, functional and positive.

HEAD INJURY AND RESPITE CARE

This need for support and respite care is due to the fact that
families living a head injury experience are challenged by a long-term

situation which may last a life time. This is a stark contrast to acute illness which has a built-in respite due to a time limitation as compared to the expanding and long-term demands of chronic conditions which can intensify the need for respite care.

Also, there is an added stressor for families when a family member's behavior becomes destructive, aggressive and dangerous. This occurs when the person changed by head injury is perceived as a stranger whose behavior makes an out-of-home placement attractive and home care more problematic. An explanation for this reaction is that families are so burdened and frustrated that they "burnout", and make alternate living arrangements, not by choice, but out of frustration and desperation. One problem common to families living a head injury experience is the reluctance to seek help until they are at the point of physical, financial and emotional exhaustion, as Waaland and Kreutzer (1988) state:

> Prolonged use of maladaptive coping strategies and persistent feelings of helplessness are related to patient confusion, marital conflict, and parental overprotection or inconsistencies. (p.57)

Often, at this point, great damage has been done and a comprehensive intervention program must be instituted to try to stabilize the patient, as well as the family. This can be achieved through a combination of direct services as well as life and living seminars which provide information, skills, and peer support.

Not only does respite care help families to cope with the challenges of a brain injury, it also helps the person experiencing a brain injury by creating an opportunity to have their basic needs periodically met by the respite care process and in turn afford a chance for "non-maintenance interaction" with the family.

While the priority is to maintain the person in the community with their families, a problem is that all communities are not in a position to provide significant support and some families do not want to, or feel that they cannot take care of a family member.

While respite care should be a component of a comprehensive intervention, treatment and rehabilitation model, attention must be given to the multidimensional problems that families often face, such as role fatigue, stress, the need for rejuvenation and the importance of maintaining quality of life. DeJong, Batavia, and Williams (1990) address this point when they state:

> Provision of respite care cannot be addressed by the family, which needs temporary relief from the situation, nor by society, which typically is too removed from the situation to provide humane care. Respite care, and other services such as grocery shopping and housekeeping, may be provided effectively by members of the community. (p.17)

Frequently, the major stressor in the head injury experience is the dramatic change of roles. These role shifts can occur when the affectionate, responsible spouse becomes a demanding, irresponsible patient and the loving, caring wife or husband becomes a resentful caregiver with a role that is seen more as a "curse" than an opportunity. Rosenthal (1987) addresses the intensity of the situation when he states:

> Spouses may feel as though they are living with strangers; relatives may reject the injured member because they do not recognize and/or understand how to deal with subtle neurobehavioral disturbances. Friends may vanish due to the head injured patient's personality change, physical or mental limitation, impaired social skills, or inability to "fit in" with the group. (p.55)

The following examples may provide a perspective on the stressors that could warrant, require, or demand respite care:

1. A husband with head injury who cannot regulate body functions and has to be constantly supervised. Enormous stress is placed upon the wife and children because there is a six-year-old child who is severely disabled and requires a life support system.

2. The elderly parent who has a child with a severe developmental disability, who was able to manage with the help of her son until he sustained a brain injury and became a patient rather than a helper.

3. A woman who has multiple sclerosis and cannot get the help from her husband who was brain injured and is unable to provide the care she needs. This is complicated by the constant turnover of workers and lack of a supportive family.

What these examples have in common is the intensity of a situation that has resulted in increased family stress and has created the potential for accelerated familial deterioration. Respite care in such situations enables the family to create a pause in the caregiving process and develop a different frame of reference. As a result, family members are able to renegotiate their familial roles, as well as establish new ones which are more conducive to coping, rejuvenation, and survival.

CONCLUSION

A major contribution of respite care for families challenged by head injury is the ability to replace desperation with hope, nothingness with dreams, and isolation with support.

While it would be wonderful if no child, adult, or family had to deal with the ravages of head injury, life, unfortunately, does not always conform to such hopes or aspirations. When head injury occurs, it is often an unending, familial nightmare that depletes resources, insults dignity, and often pushes the family to the brink of desperation. Sometimes they survive. Other times, however, the outcome is more disappointing.

The enormity of head injury is so pervasive, powerful, and all-encompassing that coping with it cannot be the sole responsibility of the family. Therefore, it is imperative that health care professionals, as well as others, be aware of and in tune with the complexities surrounding the head injury experience and how it impacts the family. As Rosenthal and Young (1988) state:

> Failure to understand the family dynamics following head injury and to provide the appropriate intervention is likely to limit the potential success of any rehabilitation program. (p.42)

In discussing head injury, there are several concepts that should be considered:

- No person or family is completely or ever prepared for the personalized reality of a head injury experience.
- Head injury changes a family and challenges its resources.
- A head injury brings out the best and worst in people and in families.
- Head injury can deplete family resources as well as create them.
- Often the only support available is the family, by intent or by default.
- All people do not have families they can rely on.
- Not all families are capable of responding to the needs of a head injured family member.
- New skills are needed by the family to meet the ongoing challenges created by head injury.
- Not everyone is going to improve or get better.
- Sometimes the best programs do not make a difference.
- Coping with head injury is an ongoing developmental process for the patient as well as the family.
- Respite care is often the difference between coping and deteriorating.
- Not all family members love or hate the person with head injury.
- Often families survive by creating hope based upon desperation and not reality.
- Existing health care resources can help as well as hinder adjustment.

These points are made as selected examples of issues that must be expanded, explored, understood, and attended to if the family and friends of people challenged by a head injury are to renegotiate a position of survival, development, enrichment, and attainment for themselves and their family.

When discussing the differential impact of head injury, we must be aware that the resources, problems, needs, hopes, and dreams of people are as different as snowflakes. While the element of individuality is the key to emotional survival, it must be fueled by the commonality which all challenged people and their families share. This commonality is the active ingredient which can enable people to negotiate the challenges of a head injury by recognizing they are not alone and that respite care services are or should be available to them. It is most unfortunate when a person's pain and frustration is increased by the ignorance of resources and models rather than lack of them. One explanation for this lack of awareness is that in the midst of a trauma, people are so devastated that they are unable to cope with the hassles of identifying the very systems that are designed to help them.

The value of respite care and self help organizations is that they enable families to maximize their chances for survival when challenged by a head injury. Why should people in extreme need feel isolated? Can we not learn from each other, share mutual strengths, and create an environment that facilitates a reasonable quality of life?

Head injury has the power to limit those affected by it, as well as fragment the family. Respite care and human concern have the potential of putting illness, disability and head injury into perspective and creating an option for the family to live as fully as possible. In fact, head injury is not a trauma which negates humanity but rather is a life experience which gives every one a chance to demonstrate how human, caring, committed, compassionate, and realistic they are. The following personal statement, "Things Change," explore the complexity and evolution of a friendship over many years.

This chapter has been adapted from a chapter entitled "Respite Care: A Vehicle for Hope, the Buffer Against Desperation," in Family Interventions Throughout Chronic Illness and Disability. By Dell Orto, A.E., Power, P.W., and Gibbons, M. (Springer, 1988).

Personal Statement

THINGS CHANGE
(A Friend's Perspective)

Michelle was born before her mother completed her college degree, and two sons followed soon after. Both boys were behavioral problems at school, partially due to learning disabilities and possible attention deficit disorders. The family valued education and both parents were very involved in their children's academic development. They pushed the school system to provide specialized teaching services for their boys. The parents both recognized that their boys were bright, and had hopes for them being successful in school. Their daughter was doing very well in school. The parents were also involved in all aspects of their children's lives.

Michelle's parents were distant from their own families, and, beginning with sons' difficulties in school, adopted an us-against-them attitude toward people outside the family. The boys continued to get into trouble outside the home both in school and with the police for minor antics. The parents were always willing to defend their sons and neither son hesitated to turn to their parents for help. Their daughter continued to do well in school and stay out of trouble with the police, although she had adopted a fearless attitude toward authority figures after witnessing her parents defend her brothers many times.

Months after graduating from school, Michelle was severely injured while she was a passenger on a motorcycle. Initially there was little hope for her survival. She had extensive internal injuries and a severe head injury. When it became more certain that she would live, there was very little hope that she would be able to function in any way. During the acute phase of the injury, the parents had an around-the-clock vigil at Michelle's bedside. Her mother left her job in order to stay at the hospital full-time. At no time did either parent ask family or friends for help, instead rejecting help from friends when it was offered. In the eyes of many they were hyper-functional and very capable to manage all their affairs. The boys suffered greatly by the impact of their sister's injuries and the absence of their parents, and began to get into more trouble with the local police. The older son had been using drugs recreationally for many years and his drug use increased.

Michelle remained in the acute phase of her injuries for almost a year. She suffered many complications. During this year, people who had been friends with the parents never saw nor heard from them and all offers of help were politely rejected. It was determined that Michelle would go to a rehabilitation hospital while she was still on a ventilator. Because of the extent of her head and spinal cord injuries, it was certain that she would never walk. She would have very limited control over her arms. Possibly she would learn to speak again, but only after intensive speech therapy. While Michelle was in the rehabilitation hospital her parents visited every day, but they no longer remained at her bedside round-the-clock. Their anxiety had been soothed by a speech therapist who had taken the time to answer their questions and address their concerns. At this point, Michelle's mother was able to return to work part-time and spend some time with her youngest son. The family continued to reject help from friends, but began to attend some social functions. Michelle remained in the rehabilitation hospital for eighteen months during which time her parents prepared their home for her return. Michelle was quadriplegic, with a spastic paralysis, had severe cognitive difficulties, and spoke incomprehensively. Michelle's brother was very much against Michelle's homecoming. He feared the loss of his parents again, and was furious with Michelle because of her disabilities. Again, Michelle's mother left work to be with him. She learned all the nursing skills needed to care for Michelle and her husband helped with all the heavy tasks of lifting and bathing.

Michelle had been home for over three years when her mother suffered a nearly fatal heart attack. For many years, her mother had been cautioned to take care of herself and her heart condition. The heart attack forced her to give up some of the care she had been providing. Following the heart attack, Michelle hired personal care attendants to provide her with her physical needs. During the two years that Michelle had been home, her speech and cognitive abilities improved while her physical disabilities remained the same. Although her family had often rejected outside help, Michelle welcomed it. She had always been a very social person and she struggled to rebuild a social life. This rebuilding began with the hiring of personal care attendants. The first hired was a woman she had been friendly with in high school. Together, with the P.C.A., Michelle began to get out of the house more often. She began to struggle for independence from her mother who, although she was unable to provide much of the physical care, wanted to spend all her time with Michelle. Michelle wanted to be able to build a life for herself that included partying with friends her own age. It was now six years since the accident and few of Michelle's friends came around anymore. Michelle struggled to gain acceptance but was unable to run with the crowd she had socialized with before the accident. Michelle's speech was still very difficult to understand and she continued to have cognitive difficulties which caused her friends great discomfort.

Nine years after the accident, her mother died of a massive stroke at age fifty-three. The boys, both of whom had been outside the family for years, returned for the funeral. After years of isolation, the funeral brought family and friends together. Both sons moved back into town shortly after their mother's death. Michelle continued to get most of her needs met by paid professional staff instead of family members. Two years later, her father remarried and his new wife was willing to help the family with Michelle's needs.

Today, Michelle complains of feeling lonely because of the absence of past friends. Her older brother spends more time with her these days. She manages some of her feelings of grief and anger by using drugs and alcohol that her brother supplies for her. She states that getting high really helps when she feels low. She doesn't see her drug use as a problem and because she is unable to get her own supply and administer her own dose, she doesn't see it as a potential problem either. Television is a constant companion. She states that she is addicted to the soap operas. Michelle never watched television before her injury and believed that most of the shows were written for idiots. She used to love to read but no longer knows how. Recently she was turned on to books on tape and she enjoys these a great deal. Michelle is able to ask for help and attempts to stay connected with others outside of her family.

Thinking back, I must admit that there were years that I didn't visit Michelle at all. The times I did visit were very difficult for me. First of all the visits always took place in her parents' home. Before the accident, we never spent any time together in our parents' homes. I felt even more uncomfortable now because I believed that her parents were angry with me for not visiting more often, and because I reminded them of Michelle before the accident. I never knew what to talk about when I was there. I didn't want to talk about my life and all the things that I was doing because Michelle could do none of these things. Michelle's personality seemed changed. She was no longer mischievous. Earlier in our friendship, I admired her ability to create fun in almost every situation, and her sense of adventure.

One afternoon, about seven years after the accident, I was visiting with Michelle while her mother was out of the house. As soon as her mother left the house, Michelle asked me if I wanted to smoke some pot. We did, and drank a few beers. We had a lot of fun that afternoon. Afterwards, I worried about whether or not it was okay that we partied together. Before the accident, Michelle and I drank every time we were together and now, while I wanted her to feel good and have fun, I worried about the effects of drinking and drugging on her health. Shortly after that day, I entered treatment for my own addiction problems and didn't see Michelle for a couple of years after that. Now when we get together, usually over holidays, we talk about our growing families, our nieces and nephews. Being an aunt is one thing that we have in common and it's a source of joy for both of us.

The years of isolation might have been avoided if the family had been able to trust in the assistance of the helping professionals. Because of their difficulty with trust even before the accident, it would have taken extraordinary sensitivity on the part of the team working with the family. After years of isolation and chaos, the family is able to function reasonably well today. The boys both have families today, and they are very involved with their sister and father. Michelle loves being an aunt; she spends most of her money on clothes and toys for her nephews and niece. She is learning to read again and spends a lot of time reading the children's books to them. She has a role in the family again that gives her life purpose and meaning.

Today my relationship with Michelle is more comfortable than it has been in the 15 years since the accident. She continues to get better slowly and we can spend quality time together, boasting about our nieces and nephews. For years I had difficulty knowing what to talk about because I feared anything I could talk about in my life would remind her of her loss. The family was somewhat hostile toward me for years because I didn't visit often enough. I reminded the parents of what they had hoped for for Michelle. They are no longer angry, and it is much easier to visit the family home. They are working their way through their loss and are able to manage the grief that they continue to experience. In almost every way, the family is a functional unit who care for each other and help each other weather the difficulties of life as it is and the loss of their dreams, how they wanted it to be. I guess things change.

Discussion Questions on the Personal Statement "Things Change: A Friend's Perspective"

1. How does managing and advocating for children who have behavioral problems prepare or not prepare parents to cope with a child with a brain injury?

2. How does the fact that Michelle was injured on a motorcycle influence the coping of the parents?

3. Is surviving an accident with little hope for recovery a burden or challenge to this family?

4. What is your reaction to the statement, "Parents had an around-the-clock vigil at Michelle's bedside."?

5. How can help be offered when families do not want it?

6. How can siblings who "suffer greatly" be supported during the treatment and rehabilitation process?

7. What are the issues and complications generated by Michelle having a head injury and a spinal cord injury?

8. What response would be helpful for Michelle's brother since he did not want to be displaced by her?

9. What are the issues generated by Michelle's mother's near fatal heart attack?

10. Why did the death of Michelle's mother "bring the family together"?

11. Is Michelle's use of drugs a problem?

12. If your best friend was in a situation similar to Michelle's, how long would you want to or be able to maintain a relationship? Five, ten, 15 years?

SET 15

HOW CAN I HELP?

Perspective: A characteristic of most suffering is that it is done alone. This is especially true when families are forced to retreat from society and focus all of their energy on the caregiving process. A major tenent of respite care is that the more a burden is shared, the more bearable it becomes.

Exploration:
1. Do you know a family dealing with a head injury. Have you considered reaching out and providing support?
2. Would you respond differently if the patient was a child?
3. If you belong to a religious organization, can you identify how this religious organization demonstrates the principle of becoming involved like the good samaritan by taking care of people in this life as well as the next.

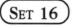

SET 16

WHO NEEDS THIS KIND OF HELP?

Perspective: When families are in a state of crisis, they need to be listened to, responded to, and treated with sensitivity, caring and respect. Often, the stress of health care and rehabilitation environments creates a situation in which professional and nonprofessional staff do not provide help but rather create pain by insensitive and non-helpful remarks.

Exploration: List from your personal and/or professional frame of reference examples of how health care and human service professionals have been helpful in dealing with the impact of a head injury.

Helpful Responses:
(example: It is not easy but we will be there to help.)
1.
2.
3.
4.
5.

Not Helpful Responses:
(example: After all, your daughter was an alcoholic who should not have been driving.)
1.
2.
3.
4.
5.

ADDITIONAL DISCUSSION QUESTIONS

1. Who should provide respite care in your community?

2. Should respite care be paid for by insurance?

3. Should families be financially compensated for the home care of a family member with a brain injury?

4. What would you consider adequate respite care for a family who has a five-year-old child with a brain injury and a parent with terminal cancer?

5. List the important components of a respite care program designed to meet the needs of families challenged by a head injury.

6. Should individuals or families be "legally" forced to provide respite care for a family member?

7. What would be your reaction to a proposal that suggested that all religious facilities should have as part of their mission the provision of respite care services for the community?

8. How would you challenge the position that respite care is a luxury and should not be considered an integral part of a discharge plan?

9. What are the criteria you would use to decide if a family needed respite care?

REFERENCES

Armstrong, C. (1991, June). Emotional changes following brain injury: Psychological and Neurological components of depression, denial and anxiety. *Journal of Rehabilitation*, pp. 14-17.

Botuck, S., & Winsberg, B. G. (1991). Effects of respite on mothers of school-age and adult children with severe disabilities. *Mental Retardation, 29*(1), 43-47.

Brown, B. W., & McCormick, T. (1988). Family coping following traumatic head injury: An exploratory analysis with recommendations for treatment. *Family Relations, 37*, 12-16.

Campbell, C. H. (1988). Needs of relatives and helpfulness of support groups in severe head injury. *Rehabilitation Nursing, 13*(6), 320-325

Cohen, S., & Warren, R. (1985). *Respite care*. Austin, TX: Pro Ed.

DeJong, G., Batavia, A. I., & Williams, J. M. (1990). Who is responsible for the lifelong well-being of a person with a head injury? *Journal of Head Trauma, 5*(1), 9-22.

Dell Orto, A. E. (1988). Respite care: A Vehicle for hope, the buffer against desperation. In P. W. Power, A. E. Dell Orto, & M. Gibbons (Eds.), *Family interventions throughout chronic illness and disability*. Springer, 1988.

Durgin, C. J. (1989, May/June). Techniques for families to increase their involvement in the rehabilitation process. *Cognitive Rehabilitation*, pp. 22-25.

Graff, S., & Minnes, P. (1989). Stress and coping in caregivers of persons with traumatic head injuries. *Journal of Applied Social Sciences, 13*(2), 293-316.

Grant, G., & McGrath, M. (1990). Need for respite-care services for caregivers of persons with mental retardation. *American Journal of Mental Retardation, 94*(6), 638-648.

Hegeman, K. M. (1987). A care plan for the family of a brain trauma client. *Rehabilitation Nursing, 13*(5), 254-258.

Jarman, D. J., & Stone, J. A. (1989, May/June). Brain injury: Issues and benefits arising with a family support group. *Cognitive Rehabilitation*, pp. 30-32.

Lawton, M. P., Brody, E. M., Saperstein, A., & Grimes, M. (1989). Respite services for caregivers: Research findings for service planning. *Home Health Care Services Quarterly, 10*(1/2), 5-32.

Marks, R. (1987). The family dimension in long term care: An assessment of stress and intervention. *Pride Institute Journal of Long Term Home Health Care, 6*(2), 18-25.

Oddy, M., Humphrey, M., & Uttley, D. (1978). Stresses upon the relatives of head-injured patients. *British Journal of Psychiatry, 133*, 507-513.

Pearson, M. A., & Deitrick, E. P. (1989). Support for family caregivers: A volunteer program for in-home respite care. *Caring, 3*(12), 18-20, 22.

Pullo, M. L., & Hahn, S. (1979). *Respite care: A family support service*. Madison, WI: United Cerebral Palsy of Wisconsin, Inc.

Ridley, B. (1989). Family response in head injury: Denial ... or hope for the future? *Soc. Sci. Med., 29*,(4), 555-561.

Rimmerman, A. (1989). Provision of respite care for children with developmental disabilities: Changes in maternal coping and stress over time. *Mental Retardation, 27*(2), 99-103.

Rosenthal, M. (1987). Traumatic head injury: Neurobehavioral consequences. In B. Caplan (Ed.), *Rehabilitation psychology desk reference* (pp.37-63). Rockville, Aspen.

Rosenthal, M., & Young, T. (1988). Effective family intervention after traumatic brain injury: Theory and practice. *Journal of Head Trauma Rehabilitation, 3*(4), 42-50.

Stroker, R. (1983). Impact of disability on families of stroke clients. *Journal of Neurosurgical Nursing, 15*, 6:360-365.

Waaland, P. K., & Kreutzer, J. S. (1988). Family response to childhood traumatic brain injury. *Journal of Head Trauma Rehabilitation, 3*(4), 51-63.

Zeigler, E. A. (1989, May/June). The importance of mutual support for spouses of head injury survivors. *Cognitive Rehabilitation*, pp. 34-37.

11

ALCOHOL AND DISABILITY: A HEAD INJURY PERSPECTIVE

11

Alcohol And Disability:
A Head Injury Perspective

Perspective

Alcohol use and abuse causes illness, violence, accidents, disability, death and a variety of other problems for individuals, families and society (Abel & Ziendenberg, 1985; Anda, Williamson, & Remington, 1988; Bratter & Forrest, 1985; Fallon, 1990; Hingson & Howland, 1987; Huth, Maier, Simnowitz, & Herman, 1983; Jones, 1989; Kinney & Leaton, 1987; Kirkpatrick & Pearson, 1978; Kreutzer, Myers, Harris, & Zasler, 1990; Levin, Benton, & Grossman, 1982; Lowenstein, Weissberg, & Terry, 1990; Luna, Maier, Souder, et al., 1984; Noble, 1978; Shipley, Taylor, & Falvo, 1990; Soderstrom & Cowley, 1987; Teplin, Abram, & Stuart 1989; Waller, 1990; Yates, Meller, & Toughton, 1987). Not only is this a tragedy for all involved, it is an ongoing shame that our society encourages, condemns, but also tends to ignore!

Concern about alcohol and its effects was expressed more than 100 years ago as reflected in the following quote by Blair (1888) from *The Conflict Between Man and Alcohol*:

> The conflict between man and alcohol is as old as civilization, more destructive than any other form of warfare, and as fierce to-day [sic] as at any time since the beginning.
>
> It is not an exaggeration to say that no other evil known in human history has been of such vast proportions and lamentable consequences as that of alcoholic intemperance. As the whole past of the race has been cursed by it, so its whole future is threatened with increasing calamity, unless there be a period put to its ravages.

> It is a peculiarity of this curse that it is developed by civilization, and then, like the parricide, it destroys the source of its own life.
>
> But although alcohol is his special foe, it by no means confines its dagger and chalice to civilized man. Combining with the spirit of a mercenary commerce, this active essence of evil is hunting and extirpating the weaker races and indigenous populations of uncivilized countries from the face of the earth. (p.ix)

These timeless thoughts capture and reflect several issues that are central in a discussion of alcohol and its relation to disability and head injury.

The common themes are that::

- there is a war going on that has more victims than most conflicts of recent memory
- the ravages of alcohol-induced illness, disability and head trauma are complex, long-lasting and often irreversible
- the forces of alcohol destruction are often driven by profit and commercial interests at the expense of the common good
- certain people are very vulnerable to the promise of alcohol due to their pre-trauma or post-trauma cognitive, physical and emotional deficits

The problem for many individuals and families challenged by alcohol is intensified when they realize that there are forces in our society which have the power to impair, maim and kill their children, friends, strangers, spouses, parents and themselves. A direct result of this reality is the pervasive helplessness most people feel in controlling their destiny as well as the well-being of their loved ones.

An additional consideration in a discussion of alcohol and its relationship to disability and head trauma is how a family uses or abuses alcohol. If a family's alcohol use is casual, there may be a negative reaction when the effects of alcohol abuse by a family member conflict with familial value systems and traditions. Frequently alcohol use is condoned by the family because it considers alcohol as recreational and less harmful than "illegal drugs." This tolerant position can change dramatically if under the influence of alcohol, a loved one is involved in a vehicular accident and becomes disabled or brain injured. It is within this transition from alcohol use to irreparable harm that most families find their ultimate agony, pain, sorrow, and regrets.

The harsh reality is that alcohol use and abuse will and does create personal and familial stress because illness, disability and head injury are direct and indirect consequences of it.

When discussing alcohol it must be kept in mind that alcohol is a drug and, as Fort (1973) stated, our most dangerous drug:

... alcohol is our most widely used mind-altering drug. It is by far
our hardest drug and constitutes our biggest drug problem in that
it kills, disables, addicts, and makes psychotic more people than
all the other drugs put together. (p.v-vi)

ALCOHOL AND DISABILITY

There has been an increased awareness of the problems related to
substance abuse by persons living with illness and disability, as well as
the role of alcohol as a cause of disability and a major impediment in
treatment and rehabilitation (Beck, Marr, & Taricone, 1991; Benshoff &
Leal, 1990; Boros, 1989; Cherry, 1988; Dean, Fos, & Jensen, 1985;
Frieden, 1990; Glass, 1981; Gorski, 1980; Greenwood, 1984; Greer, 1986;
Hadley, 1982; Hindman & Widem, 1981; Heinemann, Keen, Donahue,
& Schnoll, 1988; Heinemann, Doll, & Schnoll, 1989; Krause, 1992;
Kirubakaran, Kuman, Powell, Tyler, & Armatas, 1986; Lowenstein,
Weissberg, & Terry, 1990; Moore & Seigel, 1989; O'Donnell, Cooper,
Gessner, Shehan, & Ashley, 1982; O'Farrell, Connors, & Upper, 1983;
Pires, 1989; Rasmussen & DeBoer, 1981; Rohe & Depompolo, 1985;
Straussman, 1985; Waller, 1990; Woosley, 1981).

When disability is conceptualized as a loss of control over one's
physical or emotional destiny, the stage is set for some individuals to
cope with the concomitant stress, pain, grief and depression by initiating or increasing their use of and dependency on alcohol and other
drugs (Frisbie & Tun, 1984; Woosley, 1981).

The irony of the substance abuse process is that even though it has
resulted in a severe disability, some individuals may still rely on drugs
and alcohol to cope with their physical and/or emotional loss (Greer,
1986; Greer, Roberts, & Jenkins, 1990). However, it is important to
consider that, among persons living with a disability, there are those
individuals who had a problem with substance abuse prior to the
disability, as well as those persons who began using alcohol or other
drugs following the onset of a disability.

ROLE OF ALCOHOL IN HEAD INJURY

Recently increased attention has been given to the relationship
between alcohol and head injury (Alterman & Tarter, 1985; Blackerby
& Baumgarten, 1990; Bond, 1986; Burke, Weselowski, & Guth, Jernigan,
1991; Jones, 1989; Kreutzer, Doherty, Harris, & Zasler, 1990; Kreutzer,
Marwitz, & Wehman, 1991; Langley & Kiley, 1992; Miller, 1989;
Peterson, Rothfleisch, Zelazo, & Pihl, 1990; Rimel, Giordani, Barth,
Boll, & Jane, 1981; Rimel, Giordani, Barth, & Jane, 1982; Rimel, 1982;
Ruff et al., 1990; Ryan & Butters, 1983; Solomon & Sparadeo, 1992;
Sparadeo & Gill, 1989; Sparadeo, Strauss, & Barth, 1990; Sparadeo,
Strauss, & Kapsales, 1992; Tobis, Puri, & Sheridan, 1982, NHIF, 1988).

In a very timely and relevant article entitled *"Alcohol, Brain Injury, Manslaughter and Suicide."*, Kreutzer, Myers, Harris and Zasler (1990) articulate the relationship between alcohol and head injury. The opening line of this article states:

> Evidence clearly indicates there are interrelationships between alcohol use, risk for brain injury, and post-injury psychosocial adjustment. (p.14)

A similar point is made by Seaton and David (1990):

> For the individual with TBI, substance abuse has a profoundly destructive influence. There is an increase not only in the risk of reinjury, but also in the aggravation of cognitive deficits and poor impulse control, and a diminution of social skills. (p.44)

The complexity of the problem and the synergistic relationship between alcohol and traumatic brain injury is summarized by Langley (1991) in a literature review related to the causal role of alcohol in the acquisition of traumatic brain injury as well as its deleterious effect on rehabilitation. Langley concludes:

* Alcohol use involved in the acquisition of 35 to 66 percent of all traumatic brain injuries.
* Alcohol is also a key factor in the failure of community reintegration efforts for many clients.
* Alcohol detrimentally affects functions associated with the prefrontal and temporal lobes including memory, planning, verbal fluency, complex motor control, and the modulation of emotionality.
* Alcohol use may further reduce the capacity for behavioral self-regulation for those clients who have compromised prefrontal-temporal functioning due to traumatic brain injury.

These observations present a harsh reality for persons and families who must adjust to initial losses related to alcohol use and live with its ongoing consequences.

In discussing why head injury survivors turn to alcohol Sparadeo et al. (1990) state:

> Head injury survivors are particularly vulnerable to use of alcohol or other substances during or after the rehabilitation process, for several reasons. They must deal with the losses experienced following the injury. They are often alienated by their peers and treated differently by family members. Activity levels are often curtailed, and a significant degree of boredom is a common experience. This combination of factors contributes greatly to the use of substances, particularly alcohol. (p.3)

DUAL DIAGNOSIS

While families and individuals are faced with the often complex and demanding consequences of head injury, there is an added stress when alcohol and substance abuse results in a multidimensional disability and presents a unique set of problems related to dual diagnosis.

The long term consequences of and limited treatment resources for head injured substance abusers is discussed by Sparadeo et al. (1990):

> It is becoming more common to see addicted or severely troubled substance abusers several years after a head injury. These individuals are usually referred to a postacute head injury rehabilitation facility or a substance abuse program. Unfortunately, treatment opportunities for these dual diagnosis cases are very limited. (p.4)

The importance of dual diagnosis related to mental illness and substance abuse is addressed by Pepper and Ryglewicz (1984), Ramsey, Vredenburgh and Gallagher (1983), Brown and Backer (1988); Carey (1989), Daley, Moss and Campbell (1987) Kofoed, Kania, Walsh and Atkinson (1986), McKelvy, Kane and Kellison (1987), Brown, et al (1989), and Sternberg (1986). The challenging reality for families of persons who are mentally ill is that they are often overwhelmed by the demands and problems associated with the primary diagnosis of mental illness. Consequently, they may not be concerned about, aware of, or able to cope with the potential problems associated with the synergistic effects of mental illness and alcohol abuse which could result in a physical disability such as head injury. The potential for this to occur is clarified when suicide attempts are related to mental illness complicated by substance abuse. It is important to realize that if a suicide attempt is not successful, there may still be irreversible physical and emotional consequences for the patient and the family. An example of this is poignantly illustrated by the case of a young man who had a history of mental illness and alcohol abuse. He attempted suicide by jumping from a building. He survived with a severe head injury complicated by a spinal cord injury. This was an overwhelming tragedy for the family which was focussing on the long-term demands of a psychiatric disorder and a substance abuse problem and was not prepared for the additional demands of traumatic brain injury complicated by a quadriplegia.

SITUATIONAL VARIABLES

When discussing disability, head injury and alcohol use, it is important to consider the many situational variables related to the overall experience. For example:

- Was the injured person an alcohol or substance abuser prior to the accident?
- Did alcohol have a role in the situation?
- Was the injured person in "control" or a victim (e.g., driver or passenger)?
- Was the person a non-substance user who was a victim of a drunk driving situation? A crime of violence?
- Prior to the trauma, was alcohol part of the families lifestyle?
- Are alcohol and other drugs a threat to treatment and rehabilitation due to resumption of use or initiation of dependency?

While the legal drug, alcohol, has had a major impact on a person's life, it does not mean that the problem has been eliminated for the person or the family. This point is illustrated by the fact that some people who have sustained an alcohol-related head injury or spinal cord injury may still drink and/or drink and drive and continue to place themselves and their families at risk.

The importance of this point is that there are stressors and residuals consequent to alcohol abuse which can be far more problematic than the alcohol abuse alone. The following case synopsis further illustrates this point:

> A person was referred for treatment with the presenting problem of adjusting to his disability. During the initial evaluation, a complex familial situation emerged. Prior to his injury, the individual was engaged in a problematic marital situation which involved alcohol abuse. The day the couple decided to obtain a divorce, the husband, while intoxicated, was severely head injured as a result of an industrial accident. He was comatose for three months and, after a year of hospitalization and rehabilitation, he still had major cognitive difficulties and physical limitations. The harsh reality was that the complexity of the situation and financial considerations forced the couple to live together amidst an affective environment clouded by anger, bitterness and resentment. Just as alcohol was part of the pre-injury lifestyle, it became more of a problem during rehabilitation. This was manifested in physical and emotional abuse which culminated in legal action to charges of mutual assault and physical injury to the wife resulting in a complex physical, emotional and legal situation.

Another case synopsis which illustrates the compounding nature of the effects of alcohol abuse is as follows:

> A young woman sought out treatment for the presenting problem of chronic alcohol abuse and concern about her marriage. During treatment, her husband expressed his intentions to file for a divorce. When this occurred, the client, while under the influence of alcohol, went out for a drive and crashed

> into a tree. She sustained severe head trauma, was facially
> disfigured, lost sight in one eye and needed many surgical
> procedures related to her broken hips and legs. Her husband
> promised not to seek the divorce if she would sign all of their
> assets over to him. When this occurred, he left the country and
> left her destitute and suicidal. When asked about his actions he
> stated he did not want to be married to a cripple.

Both these case summaries reflect the enormity and complexity of the disability experience for couples who are stressed by a physical and emotional realities complicated by alcohol use. In both cases, the marital system was problematic prior to the head injury and collapsed when the added stress of the head injury experience took an additional toll. However, it must be pointed out that there are occasions when a dysfunctional marital or familial system can improve if it can respond to the challenges of a disability by initiating new behaviors and establishing more functional roles. This occurred in the following case synopsis:

> A young couple who had been married for five years were on the
> verge of a separation. This situation was a result of several years
> of individual alcohol abuse and domestic violence. The result
> was that the couple lived in the same house but led very separate
> lives. They had two children whom they both cared for. One
> evening the young woman was in an alcohol-related accident
> which was life-threatening and was complicated by a head
> injury. Her husband responded to the crisis by stopping his
> drinking, organizing the family and becoming invested in the
> well being and rehabilitation of his wife. A year later, they both
> were alcohol-free, intact as a family, and were appreciative of the
> gains that were a direct result of trauma and loss. The young man
> said it best when he stated "I guess our lives were so out of control
> and distorted by alcohol that we both needed something serious
> to happen to get our attention."

For some families, their lives are complicated by the reality that they must be vigilant in their efforts to eliminate the disastrous consequences of the legal drug alcohol, while often being forced into roles and situations that are complicated at best. The challenge is not only to cope with a head injury but also live with the losses related to poor choices and often irreversible consequences. This situation is further complicated by the fact that at any time during the life span, families can be forced into caregiver, supportive or custodial roles that they find stressful, demanding and frustrating.

In attempting to negotiate this complex process, families are often faced with the reality of their loss and the limitation of their resources. As a result, the nuclear family may feel powerless in a nuclear age.

Contributing to this powerlessness is the media which has created norms slanted more toward the hedonistic lifestyle made attainable by alcohol use. On a daily basis, children, adolescents and adults are barraged by advertisements which create the image that alcohol is a vehicle to self-fulfillment, enjoyment and excitement when in reality it is a potential short cut to brain injury, trauma, chaos, coma management, death and familial collapse. This point is made by Miller (1989) when he states:

> One need hardly comment on the glorification of life in the fast lane that deluges us in this country through advertising and the media, for example, TV beer commercials. No surprise, then, that impulsivity, drinking, driving and head injury all go together so frequently in the United States, as well as elsewhere. (p.28)

When discussing problems related to aggressive behavior following head injury, Miller (1990) states:

> The situation may be further compounded by the high rate of alcohol and drug abuse typically found in this group - substance abuse acting both as a causal factor in the injury itself (e.g., auto and industrial accidents), and as a postconcussion complication in lowering the seizure threshold or further exacerbating disinhibition in a frontally-compromised individual. (p.16)

VIOLENCE

No discussion of alcohol use is complete without attending to its relationship to violence and its consequences. Shapiro (1982) discussed the relationship between alcohol and family violence and indicated that family members are often the direct victims of violence resulting in trauma and disability. In addition to acts of physical abuse such as wife battering, there are often the long-term consequences such as head trauma which may be a direct or indirect consequence of alcohol-induced violence which occurs by intent or by default. Unfortunately, these situations often result in unforgettable realities that can be more consuming to the family than the successful rehabilitation of the abusing family member who caused the head injury of a loved one.

CONCLUSION

The awesome power of alcohol abuse is a realistic threat which may consume its victims and create a state of loss, failure, and helplessness. A person may die, be psychologically fragmented, be imprisoned by a head injury, and be the cause of a variety of personal and/or familial tragedies. In attempting to control these realities, families are faced with the task of self examination, self-exploration, and often self-incrimination as they attempt to define their role either as part of the problem or as part of the solution.

The challenge in working with persons and families challenged by a head injury and the ongoing consequences of alcohol is to begin to mobilize those resources and supports which can be stabilizing factors during an ongoing rehabilitation process.

To focus on the future benefits of treatment and rehabilitation without the development of viable alternatives to alcohol use is ignoring the potential vulnerability of this population and the potential role of alcohol in the person's life. This is a very important issue because an individual who makes a commitment to treatment and rehabilitation often assumes that there is a chance to survive and attain a reasonable quality of life. If the skills are not generalizable to the real world, relapse becomes a reality and those responsible for the design and expectations of the head injury treatment and rehabilitation process must bear the burden of failure and not project blame onto the deficits of the clients. This point is particularly relevant when referring to the person with a head injury who must continue to meet the challenges of the life and living process without alcohol use, its concomitant pathology and often irreversible consequences. As Langley (1991) states:

> For TBI clients, however, an accurate appraisal of the harmfulness of drinking may be difficult due to damage to those areas of the brain which subtend perception and understanding. The client seems unable to call to mind any negative consequences. Positive expectancies for the benefits of alcohol are often more resilient, and in the face of failure to cope with high-risk situations, could reduce motivation to abstain. (p.256)

While there are many important issues related to the treatment and rehabilitation of persons living with a head injury, there are also important issues related to the role of alcohol as a cause of illness, disability, head trauma, loss and death. How can we be content with our position as a society which reacts to the problems consequent to alcohol use but ignores the facts and minimizes the reality?

Until we acknowledge and respond to the pervasive and causal role alcohol plays in the creation of illness, disability and head trauma, we are doomed to be victims of a double standard that decries the by-products of alcohol abuse but revels in the illusion of media distortion that presents people with a dream and delivers a nightmare.

The following personal statement, "Attitude is Everything," poignantly illustrates the life-altering reality when drinking and driving results in brain damage, loss, and ongoing emotional trauma which is made bearable by having reasonable goals and a positive attitude.

PERSONAL STATEMENT

ATTITUDE IS EVERYTHING
(A Father's Perspective)

Life sure deals some unexpected cards. I was convinced that I had gotten through the rough times in my life. After I married my second wife, life seemed like it was almost perfect. She and her two boys and I and my son were becoming a real happy family until the day that tragedy struck us. This woman who had been to a retirement party where she drank too much, got behind the wheel of a car, plowed into my son and almost killed him. The doctors in the trauma center said he would live but we should start looking for nursing homes because his brain damage would cause him to be a vegetable. Whey do they say things like that? I figure they don't really know but they want to prepare you for the worst, so you won't be shocked. When I think about it, I still get mad. It's a good thing that we didn't listen to them.

My first wife and I had my son when I was 21 so when he had his accident two years ago when he was 19, I was only 40, and my second wife was 35. Her boys were younger of course, but we were definitely out of the baby-sitting stage. The point is we were still young and pretty free to do what we wanted without having to worry about the kids all the time.

After the accident, that changed. We had a "child" that needed to be watched constantly at first. After a while, we kind of tested him to see if we could leave him alone for longer periods of time. It wasn't a big problem because we're a family that has always done things together, so on the weekends we all worked on the house that we're now building on our property in Pennsylvania. During the week we had the most difficulty because both my wife and I go to work; she's a bank manager and I'm a mason. In the beginning, different people from our church would come and stay with my son. After a while, they needed to be there less and less. We're believers in the power of positive thinking. If you believe that someone can eventually be independent even when they're brain injured, you'll pass that optimistic attitude on to them; it's almost as if they breathe it in. My wife was a real independent child while she was growing up and she wouldn't let him act helpless. She kept expecting my son to take more and more responsibility. It was a little rough for her because at times she felt guilty about being hard on him, especially when the progress was slow. She went to talk to a counselor about it. She helped her see that she couldn't fix him, that he would have to fix himself, but it was okay to have expectations that eventually he would be more responsible. My wife's a backbone for this family. Sometimes I get real impatient if things move too slowly, but she convinces me that in time things will work out if we work at it. I know she's right. Even though my son's in a wheelchair most of the time, he now can stay by himself, keeps the house picked up and, a couple of times a week, he gets the dinner. The real good news is he's going back to school to learn about computers.

Before the accident, he had no ambition to have a career. All he cared about was girls and sports. He definitely was not a great student in school. Now, he still is not a great student, but he does have ambition. We know that it will be slow going. One thing about head injured people is that even if they intend to do things, they can be real slow about doing them. One minute it seems he's forgotten what he said he was going to do. That's improving because he knows that he has to do his homework or he'll be embarrassed when he goes to class. It's good because he gets to be around other people and he needs that. If you were to ask him what's the hardest thing about life after the injury, he'd say that not being able to walk is the hardest part, but if you ask me I'd say not having a normal social life is the hardest. He wants a girlfriend in the worst way and was very depressed for a long time because he thought he'd never have one. Before the accident, he was a leader type, real sure of himself and had lots of friends and girlfriends. Now, because he talks slowly and so softly, he's very self-conscious and for a long time avoided people his own age. When he was in the rehabilitation center, he met some girls who were head injured also, but I know he really wants to meet a "normal" girl. As my wife says, he was sweet before the accident and he's still that way and eventually he'll find someone who appreciates him.

I'm convinced the Lord works in strange ways. Since the accident, we're even closer as a family. The younger boys help their older brother. Of course, they fight like brothers too, but they've learned a lot of compassion. We try hard not to neglect them because of their older brother's needs; we know if we did, they'd resent him and we don't want that to happen. We haven't given up our dreams–just reorganized them. My wife was going to go to college full-time, now she'll go part-time. We were going to build our house in five years. Now we'll take ten years to build. The neat part is that it's been interesting to design a house that could accommodate a person in a wheelchair. Even if my son leaves home and lives on his own, he'll always have a comfortable home to visit. If you want something and you're willing to work hard for it, you'll get it some way. Attitude is everything.

DISCUSSION QUESTIONS ON THE PERSONAL STATEMENT "ATTITUDE IS EVERYTHING"

1. How does surviving crises and making a new beginning in life create emotional vulnerability?

2. What is an adequate sentence for a person who kills someone in a drunk driving accident? Who causes an accident that result in a head injury?

3. Do you think that the suggestion made by the doctors in the trauma center that the father should start looking for a nursing home

because their son would be a vegetable was helpful? Why or why not?

4. Discuss the impact of a head injury when it occurs at various stages of child rearing.

5. Develop a respite care program that would respond to the unique needs of this family.

6. How can the power of positive thinking be an asset, as well as a liability?

7. Discuss the positive and negative implications of the statement "My wife was a real independent child while she was growing up and she would not let him act helpless."

8. How can a head injury result in new career goals and ambition for academic as well as vocational goals?

9. Give examples of how a person with a head injury can perceive "loss" differently from parents or significant others.

10. Should individuals with a head injury be encouraged to date or marry people with a head injury as is stated in the personal statement "a normal girl"?

11. How can a head injury experience make a family closer?

12. What is meant by the statement "we haven't given up our dreams–just reorganized them"?

13. Give examples of how the concept of working hard will result in attaining a goal can provide hope, as well as frustration.

14. How are attitudes developed? How are they changed?

SET 17

ONE FOR THE ROAD

Perspective: Since many head injuries are a result of vehicular accidents, it seems reasonable to focus on the cause of the problem as well as to the effects.

One consideration is that advertising often presents alcohol use as an integral part of daily life which includes recreation, socialization and work.

Exploration: In order to better understand the scope of the issue, do the following:

1. Go through a variety of magazines and select alcohol advertisements that you think create distorted images.
2. Identify what groups of people you think would be most vulnerable.
3. Discuss the concept of "potential consequences."
4. Explore how potential consequences could be presented in the media (e.g., "This wheelchair's for you.").
5. Should advertisers, brewers, and distillers be responsible for medical costs associated with head injury consequent to drunk driving?
6. Should people with brain injuries be prevented from buying alcohol? Why/why not?
7. What disabilities are caused by alcohol?
8. What disabilities do you think could cause alcohol abuse?
9. How would you approach a person who said, "I lost so much as a result of my head injury that I need to drink just to get by."?
10. If you were brain injured, would you tend to use or abuse alcohol? What factors would influence your decision?
11. Have you ever worked with a client whose substance use undermined the treatment and rehabilitation process?
12. Should media be limited in the kind of alcohol advertising it presents to the public?
13. If you were a judge presiding over a case in which a drunk driver killed a 17-year-old and injured another 17-year-old who survived head injury, what do you think would be an appropriate sentence? What would be adequate compensation for each family?
14. What are the critical issues in the rehabilitation process which can create the conditions for substance use and abuse?
15. If a person is injured while riding a motorcycle, while under the influence of drugs or alcohol, who should be responsible for the medical costs? Should insurance be void?
16. Should the manufacturers of beer and spirits be liable for the consequences of their product?

REFERENCES

Abel, E. L., & Ziendenberg, P. (1985). Age, alcohol and violent death: A postmortem study. *Journal of Studies on Alcohol, 46*(3).

Alterman, A. I., & Tarter, R. E. (1985). Relationship between familial alcoholism and head injury. *Journal of Studies on Alcohol, 46*(3), 256-258.

Anda, R. F., Williamson, D. F., & Remington, P. O. (1988). Alcohol and fatal injuries in the U.S. *Journal of the American Medical Association, 33,* 132-147.

Beck, R., Marr, K., & Taricone, P. (1991). Identifying and treating clients with physical disabilities who had substance abuse problems. *Rehabilitation Education, 5,* 131-138.

Benshoff, J. J., & Leal, A. (1990). Substance abuse: Challenges for the rehabilitation counseling profession. *Journal of Applied Rehabilitation Counseling, 21*(3), 3.

Blackerby, W. F., & Baumgarten, A. (1990). A model treatment program for the head-injured substance abuser: Preliminary findings. *Journal of Head Trauma Rehabilitation, 5*(3), 47-59.

Blair, H. W. (1888). *The temperance movement or the conflict between man and alcohol.* Boston: William E. Smythe Company.

Bond, M. R. (1986). Neurobehavioral sequelae of closed head injury. In I. Grant & K. Adams (Eds.), *Neuropsychological assessment of neuropsychiatric disorders.* New York: Oxford University Press.

Boros, A. (Ed.) (1989). Alcohol and the physically impaired. *Alcohol Health and Research World, 13*(2), 31-36.

Bratter, T. E., & Forrest, G. G. (1985). *Alcoholism and substance abuse: Strategies for clinical intervention.* New York: The Free Press.

Brown, V. B., & Backer, T. E. (1988). The substance abusing mentally ill patient: Challenges for professional education and training. *Psychosocial Rehabilitation Journal, 12*(1), 43-54.

Brown, V. B., Ridgely, M. S., Pepper, B., Levine, I. S., & Ryglewicz, H. (1989). The dual crisis: Mental illness and substance abuse, present and future directions. *American Psychological Association, Inc. 44*(3), 565-569.

Burke, W. H., Weselowski, M. D., & Guth, W. L. (1988). Comprehensive head injury rehabilitation: An outcome evaluation. *Brain Injury, 2,* 313-322.

Carey, K. B. (1989). Emerging treatment guidelines for mentally ill chemical abusers. *Hospital and Community Psychiatry, 40,* 341-349.

Cherry, L. (1988). *Final report: Bay area project on disabilities and chemical dependency.* Available from IADD, 1034 Clubhouse Drive, Hayward, CA 94541.

Daley, D. C., Moss, H., & Campbell, F. (1987). *Dual disorders: Counseling clients with chemical dependency and mental illness.* Center City, MN: Hazelden.

Dean, J. C., Fos, A. M., & Jensen, W. (1985). Drug and alcohol use by disabled and non-disabled persons: A comparative study. *International Journal of Additions, 20,* 629-641.

Fallon, W. (1990). The effect of alcohol in the bloodstream after motor vehicle crash. *Topics in Emergency Medicine, 12*(4), 53-56.

Fort, J. (1973). *Alcohol: Our biggest drug problem and our biggest industry.* New York: McGraw-Hill.

Frieden, A. (1990). Substance abuse and disability: The role of the independent living center. *Journal of Applied Rehabilitation Counseling, 21*(3), 33-36.

Frisbie, J. H., & Tun, C. G. (1984). Drinking and spinal cord injury. *Journal of the American Paraplegic Society, 7,* 71-73.

Galbraith, S., Murray, W. R., Patel, A. R., & Knill-Jones, R. (1976). The relationship between alcohol and head injury, and its effects on the conscious level. *British Journal of Surgery, 63,* 128-130.

Glass, E. J. (1981). Problem drinking among the blind and visually impaired. *Alcohol Health and Research World, 5,* 20-25.

Gorski, R. (1980). Drug abuse and disabled people: A hidden problem. *Disabled USA, 4*(2), 8-12.

Greenwood, W. (1984). Alcoholism: A complicating factor in the rehabilitation of disabled individuals. *Journal of Rehabilitation, 72,* 51-52.

Greer, B., Roberts, R., & Jenkins, W. (1990). Substance abuse among clients with other primary disabilities: Curricular implications for rehabilitation education. *Rehabilitation Education, 4,* 33-44.

Greer, B. (1986). Substance abuse among people with disabilities: A problem of too much accessibility. *Journal of Rehabilitation, 52*, 34-38.

Hadley, R. G. (1982). Alcoholism as secondary disability: The silent saboteur in rehabilitation. *Rehab Brief: Bringing Research into Effective Focus, 6*, 1-4.

Heinemann, A. W., Keen, M., Donahue, R., & Schnoll, S. (1988). Alcohol use by persons with recent spinal cord injury. *Archives of Physical Medicine and Rehabilitation, 69*, 619-624.

Heinemann, A. W., Doll, M., and Schnoll, S. (1989). Treatment of alcohol abuse in persons with recent spinal cord injury. *Alcohol Health and Research World, 13*, 110-117.

Hindman, M., & Widem, P. (Eds.) (1981). Special issue: The multi-disabled. *Alcohol Health and Research World, 5*(1).

Hingson, R., & Howland, J. (1987). Alcohol as a risk factor for injury or death resulting from accidental falls: A review of the literature. *Journal of Studies on Alcohol, 43*(3), 212-219.

Huth, J., Maier, R., Simnowitz, D., & Herman, C. (1983). Effect of acute ethanolism on the hospital course and outcome of injured automobile drivers. *The Journal of Trauma, 23*, 494-498.

Jernigan, D. H. (1991). Alcohol and head trauma: Strategies for prevention. *Journal of Head Trauma Rehabilitation, 6*, 48-60.

Jones, G. A. (1989). Alcohol abuse and traumatic brain damage. *Alcohol Health and Research World, 13*, 104-109.

Kinney, J., & Leaton, G. (1987). *Loosening the grip: A handbook of alcohol information.* St. Louis: Times Mirror/Mosby College Publishing.

Kirkpatrick, J. B., & Pearson, J. (1978). Fatal cerebral injury in the elderly. *Journal of the American Geriatrics Society, 26*, 489-497.

Kirubakaran, V. R., Kuman, V. N., Powell, B. J., Tyler, A. J., & Armatas, P. J. (1986). Survey of alcohol and drug misuse in spinal cord injured veterans. *Journal of Studies on Alcohol, 47*, 223-227.

Kofoed, L., Kania, J., Walsh, T., & Atkinson, R. M. (1986). Outpatient treatment of patients with substance abuse and coexisting psychiatric disorders. *American Journal of Psychiatry, 143*, 867-872.

Krause, J. S. (1992). Delivery of substance abuse services during spinal cord injury rehabilitation. *Neuro Rehabilitation, 2*(1),45-51.

Kreutzer, J. S., Myers, S. L., Harris, J. A., & Zasler, W. D. (1990, July/August). Alcohol, brain injury, manslaughter and suicide. *Cognitive Rehabilitation, 8*(4), pp. 14-18.

Kreutzer, J. S., Marwitz, J., & Wehman, P. H. (1991). Substance abuse assessment and treatment in vocational rehabilitation for persons with brain injury. *Journal of Head Trauma Rehabilitation, 6*(3), 12-23.

Kreutzer, J. S., Leininger, B. E., & Harris, J. A. (1989). The evolving role of neuropsychology in community integration. In J. S. Kreutzer & P. Wehman (Eds.), *Community integration following traumatic brain injury* (pp.49-66). Baltimore: Paul H. Brookes Publishing Co.

Kreutzer, J. S., Doherty, K. R., Harris, J. A., & Zasler, N. D. (1990). Alcohol use among persons with traumatic brain injury. *Journal of Head Trauma Rehabilitation, 5*(3), 9-20.

Langley, M. J., Kiley, D. J. (1992). Prevention of substance abuse in persons with neurological disabilities. *Neuro Rehabilitation, 2*(1), 52-64.

Langley, M. J. (1991). Preventing post injury alcohol-related problems: A behavioral approach. In B. T. McMahon & L. R. Shaw (Eds.) *Work worth doing: Advances in brain injury rehabilitation* (pp.251-275). Orlando, FL: Paul M. Deutsch Press.

Langley, M. J., Lindsay, W. P., Lam, C. S., & Priddy, D. A. (1990). A comprehensive alcohol abuse treatment program for persons with traumatic brain injury. *Brain Injury, 4*(1), 77-86.

Levin, H. S., Benton, A. L., & Grossman, R. G. (1982). *Neurobehavioral consequences of closed head injury.* New York: Oxford University Press.

Lowenstein, S. R., Weissberg, M., & Terry, D. (1990). Alcohol intoxication, injuries, and dangerous behaviors, and the revolving emergency department door. *Journal of Trauma, 30*(10), 1252-1258.

Luna, G. K., Maier, R. V., Sowder, L. et al., (1984). The influence of ethanol intoxication on outcome of injured motorcyclists. *Journal of Trauma, 24*, 695-700.

McKelvy, M. J., Kane, J. S., & Kellison, K. (1987). Substance abuse and mental illness: Double trouble. *Journal of Psychosocial Nursing, 25*(1), 20-25.

Miller, L. (1989). Neuropsychology, personality and substance abuse: Implications for head injury rehabilitation. *Cognitive Rehabilitation, 7*(5), 26-31.

Miller, L. (1990, Nov./Dec.). Major syndromes of aggressive behavior following head injury: An introduction to evaluation and treatment. *Cognitive Rehabilitation*, pp. 14-19.

Moore, D. & Seigel, H. (1989). Double trouble: Alcohol and other drug use among orthopedically impaired college students. *Alcohol Health and Research World, 13*(2), 118-123.

National Head Injury Foundation (1988). *National Head Injury Foundation–Professional Council Substance Abuse Task Force White Paper.* Washington D.C.: National Head Injury Foundation.

Noble, E. P. (1978). *Alcohol and health* (Report No. HE 20.8313:2). Rockville, MD: United States Department of Health, Education, and Welfare.

O'Donnell, J. J., Cooper, J. E., Gessner, J. E., Shehan, I., & Ashley, J. (1982). Alcohol, drugs and spinal cord injury. *Alcohol Health and Research World, 6*(1), 27-29.

O'Farrell, J. J., Connors, G. J., & Upper, D. (1983). Addictive behaviors among hospitalized psychiatric patients. *Addictive Behavior, 8*, 329-333.

Pepper, B., & Ryglewicz, H. (1984). The young adult chronic patient and substance abuse. *Tie-Lines, 1*, 1-8.

Peterson, J. B., Rothfleisch, J., Zelazo, P. D., & Pihl, R. O. (1990). Acute alcohol intoxication and cognitive functioning. *Journal of Studies on Alcohol, 51*, 114-122.

Pires, M. (1989). Substance abuse: The silent saboteur in rehabilitation. *Nursing Clinics of North America, 24*(1), 291-296.

Ramsey, A., Vredenburgh, J., & Gallagher, R. M. (1983). Recognition of alcoholism among patients with psychiatric problems in a family practice clinic. *Journal of Family Practice, 17*(5), 829-832.

Rasmussen, G. A., & DeBoer, R. P. (1980/1981). Alcohol and drug use among clients at a residential vocational rehabilitation center. Special Issue. *Alcohol Health and Research World, 5*, 48-56.

Rimel, R. W. (1982). Moderate head injury: Completing the clinical spectrum of brain trauma. *Neurosurgery, 2*, 65-73.

Rimel, R. W., Giordani, B. G., Barth, J. T., & Jane, J. A. (1982). Moderate head injury: Completing the clinical spectrum of brain trauma. *Neurosurgery, 11*(3), 344-341.

Rimel, R. W., Giordani, B. G., Barth, J. T., Boll, J. B., & Jane, J. A. (1981). Disability caused by minor head injury. *Neurosurgery, 9*, 221-228.

Rohe, D. E., & Depompolo, R. W. (1985). Substance abuse policies in rehabilitation medicine departments. *Archives of Physical Medicine and Rehabilitation, 66*, 701-703.

Ruff, R., Marshall, L., Klauber, M., Blunt, B., Grant, I., Foulkes, M., Eisenberg, H., Jane, J., & Marmarou, A. (1990). Alcohol abuse and neurological outcome of the severely head injured. *Journal of Head Trauma Rehabilitation, 5*(3), 21-31.

Ryan, C., & Butters, N. (1983). Cognitive deficits in alcoholics. In B. Kissin & H. Begleiter (Eds.), *The pathogenesis of alcoholism: Biological factors.* New York: Plenum Press.

Seaton, J. D., & David, C. O. (1990). Family role in the substance abuse and traumatic brain injury rehabilitation. *Journal of Head Trauma Rehabilitation, 5*(3), 41-46.

Shapiro, R. (1982). Clinical approaches to family violence. *The family therapy collections.* Rockville: Aspen.

Shipley, R., Taylor, S., & Falvo, D. (1990). Concurrent evaluation and rehabilitation of alcohol abuse and trauma. *Journal of Applied Rehabilitation Counseling, 21*(3), 37-39.

Soderstrom, C. A., & Cowley, R. A. (1987). A national alcohol and trauma center survey. *Archives of Surgery, 122*, 1087-1071.

Solomon, D., & Sparadeo, F. R. (1992). Effects of substance use on persons with traumatic brain injury. *Neuro Rehabilitation, 2*(1), 16-26.

Sparadeo, F. R., Gill, D. (1989). Effects of prior alcohol use on head injury recovery. *Journal of Head Trauma Rehabilitation, 4*(1), 75-82.

Sparadeo, F. R., Strauss, D., & Barth, J. T. (1990). The incidence, impact and treatment of substance abuse on head trauma rehabilitation. *Journal of Head Trauma Rehabilitation, 5*(3), 1-8.

Sparadeo, F. R. Strauss, D., & Kapsales, K. B. (1992). Substance abuse, brain injury, and family adjustment. *Neuro Rehabilitation, 2*(1), 65-73.

Sternberg, D. W. (1986). Dual diagnosis: Addiction and affective disorders. *The Psychiatric Hospital, 20*, 71-77.

Straussman, J. (1985). Dealing with double disabilities: Alcohol use in the club. *Psychosocial Rehabilitation Journal, 8*(3), 8-14.

Teplin, L. A., Abram, K. M., & Stuart, K. (1989). Blood alcohol level among emergency room patients: A multivariate analysis. *Journal of Studies on Alcohol, 50*(3), 441-447.

Tobis, J. S., Puri, K. B, & Sheridan, J. (1982). Rehabilitation of the severely brain injured patient. *Scandinavian Journal of Rehabilitation Medicine, 14*, 655-667.

Waller, J. A. (1990). Management issues for trauma patients with alcohol. *Journal of Trauma, 30*(12), 1548-1553.

Weiss, R., & Frankel, R. (1989). Closed head injury and substance abuse: The dual misdiagnosis. *Professional Counselor, 3*(4), 49-51.

Woosley, E. E. (1981). Psycho-social aspects of substance abuse among the physically disabled. *Alcohol Health and Research World.* U.S. Department of Health and Human Services.

Yates, W. R., Meller, W., & Toughton, E. P. (1987). Behavioral complications of alcoholism. *American Family Physician, 35*(3), 171-175.

12

HOPE, NEED, AND REALITY

12

HOPE, NEED, AND REALITY

Head injury changes and challenges the entire family system. It often confuses the present, negates the past and distorts the future while creating opportunities for familial stress and disappointment as well as growth and development.

A primary theme of this book is that a functional family experience does not have to be negated because of the complexities and challenges of living "the head injury experience." However, to facilitate the process of learning, coping, adjusting, surviving, and living, the family needs timely and relevant interventions, appropriate skills and available support. When these needs are met, the family's reaction to and decisions about the person with a head injury can be made from a position of strength rather than by default.

Assisting families to cope with the emerging reality of a head injury is a process and not an event. It involves the efforts of health care and rehabilitation workers and significant others who are attuned to the needs of the person with a head injury, as well as the needs of the family. To expect that the family can provide support implies that the health care and rehabilitation professional is aware of the demands of adjusting to head injury, as well as the importance of assisting the family to stabilize, grow, and heal.

A harsh reality of life and living is that head injury is not rational nor is it fair! However, this statement does not limit the occurrence of a head injury experience that shatters dreams, destroys lives, changes families, and creates a complexity of health care issues that boggles the mind and rapidly depletes most resources. Given the enormity, complexity, and multidimensionality of head injury, it would be easy to concede that the problems consequent to a head injury are too overwhelming for health care and family systems with limited resources and overwhelming need. However, this complexity is the soul of the head injury movement which has set a course to meet the needs of persons and families who are living the head injury experience. The challenge facing families, victims, survivors, and health and human care providers is not a head injury problem; it is a human problem.

It is a human problem because all humans during their life experience will lose functioning and eventually die. Sometimes, there is a rational framework which facilitates the acceptance of this harsh reality. For example, older persons who have reached retirement age, have lived a fulfilling life, and have had their abilities altered by the normal conditions of life, living, and aging.

However, the deterioration of an elderly person is still a painful process, but more understandable than the randomness of most head injuries which assault the child, adolescents, and adults at the most inopportune times of their lives. This is compounded by the fact that most head injuries are often a result of human behavior which makes accepting the irreversible consequences of accidents, trauma, and irrational violence a life long challenge.

However, not everyone has the resources, support systems, or skills to negotiate a transitional process that demands acceptance of an often unpleasant reality. Fortunately, there are examples of people who have or who are surviving the life experience with the additional challenge of head injury. For the family and person challenged by and living in spite of a head injury, this is an important realization because it demonstrates that in life, there are choices: People can choose to make the best out of a most difficult situation or choose not to. But in reality is this the case? It sounds good, makes sense, but when discussing trauma, loss and disability in general or head injury in particular it is essential to realize that families are often so emotionally depleted that they may not be in a position to make choices that are in their long-term best interests. More often, decisions are made by default due to the lack of role models and skills needed to negotiate the perils, demands, and uncertainty of head injury treatment and rehabilitation.

The challenge therefore, is to present head injury from an optimistic, as well as realistic perspective. This is not an easy task because there are many myths and forces which can influence the expectations people have from the treatment and rehabilitation process. Some of these myths are:

MYTH 1: HEAD INJURY CAN BE PREVENTED

While it is a noble goal to reduce the incidence of head injury and a most important one for everyone concerned about head injury to try to attain, the reality is that no amount of education or prevention will eradicate all the variables that cause head injury (e.g., drunk driving, drug-related violence, war, accidents, sports injuries, etc.). For those persons and families challenged with head injury, the past is unalterable. The injury does exist and there is the temptation to replay that reality while hoping for a different outcome. For others who bear witness to the tragedy of head injury, there is the drive and commitment to "make sure" that this does not occur to others or to our family again.

The important point here is that we cannot prevent the inevitable, but we must try in order to be in a position to provide meaningful intervention, ongoing support, and helpful caring. However, it is critical that all interventions be based on a realistic perspective of the human condition as it is and what it will become. People are in a constant state of change, growth, and deterioration and cannot be "immunized" or isolated from the human experience. Head injury is a tragedy for all who experience it. But tragedy is an undeniable part of the human experience. Consequently, every effort should be made to help the person and family live a life of human dignity based upon human values that value life, accept mortality, and recognize vulnerability, promote hope and demonstrate caring. One of the most poignant statements a family can make is "we should have ...."

MYTH 2: RESTORATION IS MORE IMPORTANT THAN REALISTIC ACCEPTANCE

While many significant gains have been made in head injury prevention, treatment and rehabilitation, there is still a void which cannot be filled in but which must be crossed or accepted. This is the ultimate challenge for persons and families that are often faced with a choice between the ultimate sacrifice of self so that a loved one will be once again who they were, as compared to the recognition that they are who they are. It is important that at some time during the treatment and rehabilitation process that families are helped to recognize the difference between hope, hope based on desperation and hope based on reality. This is where self-help organizations and self-help groups can help develop a functional perspective for persons and families living in a twilight zone of confusion, pain, and overwhelming need.

MYTH 3: SOMEONE MUST PAY!

For many families enduring the journey of treatment and rehabilitation, this is an emotional and financial trap. Emotionally, a family may rightly feel they have been wronged. Wronged by the drunk driver whose actions place a child in a coma management program. But what if this person is uninsured, a repeat offender, or has no resources? Who or what becomes the object of attention? Is it the major television network that promotes alcohol use and abuse, manufacturers whose advertisements portray reckless driving as fun but also states, "do not drive this way"? Or is it the employer who fired a person who becomes despondent and angry and drives in a careless manner? It is at this point when families challenged by head injury are often confused and angry for the wrong reason. The issue is not who will pay, but rather what can be done to validate the person who was injured and to make the life care process more reasonable. The problem is that no amount of money can regain what was lost. No amount of money can undo the pain and sorrow, no amount of money guarantees that life will be easier or immune from other problems. While money can relieve the financial strain on a family, it can also be the cause of additional stress and strain. Consider the reaction of a family which has been awarded two million dollars in a personal injury case for their 17-year-old daughter. Two weeks later, they buy her a sports car and she becomes a quadriplegic as a result of a car accident.

An other issue is that large cash settlements have distorted the issues and created a cast system. Why should one person with traumatic brain injury have a five million dollar settlement and the best of care while another must live in squalor with a broken wheelchair and without personal care attendants because they were injured by a person without insurance? This is the real challenge of head injury treatment, intervention, and policy. To develop a system based upon human value, respect for life, and committed to family stabilization. No cost is too great if it is not at the expense of others who have too little.

MYTH 4: THE FAMILY AND PERSON WILL ALWAYS APPRECIATE MEDICAL INTERVENTION

A myth that creates stress for families is the expectation that all medical intervention is helpful and will be beneficial. However, when discussing head injury, families and health care professionals must also be able to discuss and process some very controversial emotional and unanswerable issues related to the benefit cost and effort related to intervention. For example, while some families are very happy that their family members life was saved, even though there are severe limitations, other families may not be as pleased or appreciative.

This point is well illustrated by the anger, resentment, and pain expressed by a mother who felt that the heroic efforts made a medical team on trauma helicopter did not save her child, but prevented him from dying and now has relegated him and the family to an emotional and physical prison. Apart from the financial costs, the emotional price has been individual stress and strain as well as familial chaos.

An alternative perspective is the great appreciation families have for those heroic efforts which have kept their loved one alive and have given them the chance to continue life but at a different level.

In both of these examples, there is the common element that the families are going to have to live with the consequences. The challenge for society and health care is to provide the support, encouragement, and role models needed to keep head injury in perspective and not become a ravaging force that destroys the family that is trying to survive.

CONCLUSION

It is important to realize that a common goal most people share is to make the world a better place to live within the constructs of a very individualized reality.

A major step in this process is recognizing that head injury is another component in the continued exploration of our humanity. It is not the last challenge we will face as a society, but one of many emerging realities that will test our convictions, resources, and fortitude. This point is well illustrated by the complexity of AIDS which has created great controversy for our society and health care system. If this issue is not put into perspective, how will the needs of the person who has AIDS and acquires a head trauma be treated? Or what will happen to the person and family that has been struggling to meet the needs of a head injured member who contracts AIDS? It is within a life and living perspective that many of the issues relative to head injury treatment and rehabilitation are cast into a different light or into a different darkness.

Illness, pain, head trauma, disability, loss, and death will always be with us. The tragedy is not that these aspects of the human condition occur but that if unchecked, they can, will, and do destroy the quality of life of the person challenged by head injury as well as the family cast in its shadow. The reality of head injury can never be totally eliminated but living with its consequences should be, must be, and certainly can be made more bearable!

The following personal statement, "Making Dream's Come True," captures the reality of living with a parent who was considered immortal.

PERSONAL STATEMENT

MAKING DREAMS COME TRUE
(A Son's Perspective)

All people have dreams, but few make the sacrifices to make the dreams come true. I read this written on a poster while waiting in a bus station trying to get home to see my father who was in a car accident. I wondered if I or my family had the ability to make the dream of my father's recovery a reality. To me, all of this was not quite believable or real.

My father was an immortal man of fifty who not only loved life, but also challenged it. In his lifetime, he had been wounded in Vietnam, and had recently recovered from a mild heart attack. The family believed that he could do anything he wanted to.

Our family was a high energy unit that enjoyed and celebrated life.

While I was sitting in the bus station, I wondered if there would ever be cause for celebration again. When I arrived home, I found an overwhelming situation. My in-control family was completely out of control and looking to me, as the eldest son, for support and leadership. I was not prepared for this. All I wanted was to see my father and find him getting better. Unfortunately, he was near death, on life-support, and we were thrown into a state of shock and distress. At that point, I knew that I, as well as my family, had to focus our resources and help each other survive this most difficult situation. My mother expected and needed a miracle. She was certain he would recover. I was more pessimistic, while my brothers and sisters did not know what to do.

During the long months of hospitalization, we were told that the future was uncertain and we were told to prepare ourselves for accepting small gains if they occurred. Small gains did occur, then some bigger ones. In a sense, our father emerged from the depths of the unknown and began to become connected with the world around him. This was most helpful because it was a small step in the right direction.

When dad returned home, he was in some ways his old self and in others, a new person. His role as family leader was taken over by my mother with the support of the rest of the family. The most helpful thing that happened was that all people did not abandon us. My father's employer offered my younger brothers jobs and told my father he could have a job when he got better. Even though this was unlikely, it gave us all a sense of hope.

For me and my family, the past three years have not been easy for any of us. Today, my father is living with the reality of his head injury. At times, he is very difficult to live with. He is often inflexible, pre-occupied with sports, and is compulsive about doing yard work. All in all, we are happy he is alive and wish the accident did not occur.

One thing we as a family agree; it certainly could have been worse and it may even get better.

DISCUSSION QUESTIONS ON THE PERSONAL STATEMENT "MAKING DREAMS COME TRUE"

1. How is the philosophy that "if you work hard at something, anything is possible" be helpful or distressful for families coping with a head injury?

2. What is meant by the statement "my father was an immortal man?

3. In this case, could family expectations that their father could do anything to create additional distress during rehabilitation?

4. What happens to a family when they want and need a miracle and it does not happen?

5. Discuss the employer's response to this situation. Do you think this is typical or atypical?

6. What are the characteristics of this family that have enabled it to remain cohesive during the head injury experience?

(SET 18)

TRAUMA HELICOPTER

Perspective: All families are greatly relieved when a family member survives the initial stages of a trauma and are given the opportunity to continue life. This initial relief and joy often turns to distress and sadness when a family realizes that the person they knew left them when the head injury occurred and now they are faced with the ongoing challenge of getting to know and accept a person who is a total or partial stranger. This often occurs when extraordinary and heroic efforts have less than ordinary or normal results. While not disputing the positive and miraculous outcomes of most trauma rescue flights, some have resulted in complex situations for families.

Exploration:
1. Are there situations when medical care should be withheld at the scene of an accident?
2. How would you help a family who was enraged that their child was "saved" and must spend the rest of his/her life in a coma management unit?

3. Should a hospital or its personnel be responsible for the long-term care and financial costs if they resuscitate a person without the family's approval?

(SET 19)

JUSTICE AND INJUSTICE

Perspective: In the discussion of the concept of life care plans, there are three dimensions embodied in the terminology:

*   life implies a biological component
*   care implies a beneficial interaction between people who are recipients of care and the caregivers
*   plan implies a carefully thought out sequence of decisions, acts and consequences which have short- and long-term positive benefits

In discussing life care plans for persons and families challenged by a head injury, there are other factors to be considered. They are that life may be devoid or limited in quality, that caring may be a myth driven by financial gain and that planning may be an overly detailed process which masks chaos and omits the flexibility which is needed to deal with living changing systems.

Exploration:
1. What are the essential elements of life care plans?
2. Should parents be required to return or be accountable for money awarded in settlements if they place the head injured person in a public facility?
3. Should people who receive "large" settlements be required to contribute to the care of those who were brain-injured by an uninsured driver and who are left destitute?
4. How much money represents an adequate amount for the life-long care of a brain-injured child.
5. Who should be responsible for the life long care of a severely brain-injured person if the family does not want to assume the role?
6. How much money is enough to compensate for a severe head injury? How much money is too much?
7. Can head injury be prevented?
8. Does the goal to make a person what they were prior to a head injury interfere with the acceptance of who they are post injury?
9. What are the issues generated by the treatment and rehabilitation of a person with a head injury who acquires AIDS as compared to a person with AIDS who acquires a head injury?

APPENDICES

Support Groups And State Associations Of The National Head Injury Foundation

Alabama
P.O. Box 550008
Birmingham, AL 35255
205/328-3505
800/433-8002 (Alabama only)

Arizona
1131 North Winstel Blvd.,
No. A
Tucson, AZ 85716-4022
602/326-2872
800/432-3465

Arkansas
P.O. Box 7138
Sherwood, AR 72116
501/452-7737
800/235-2443

California
8060 Florence Ave., Suite 302
Downey, CA 90240
310/803-4418

Colorado
5601 S. Broadway, Suite 350
Littleton, CO 80121
303/730-7112
800/955-2443

Connecticut
1800 Silas Deane Highway,
Suite 224
Rocky Hill, CT 06067
203/721/8111
800/669-4323 (Connecticut only)

Delaware
P.O. Box 9876
Newark, DE 19714-9876
302/654-7705

Florida
North Broward Medical Center
201 E. Sample Road
Pompano Beach, FL 33064
305/786-2400
800/992-3442 (In Florida only)
FAX: 305/786-2437

Georgia
P.O. Box 95217
Atlanta, GA 30347
404/727-5588
FAX: 404/727-5895

Hawaii
2301 B. Jasmine Street
Honolulu, HI 96816
808/732-2021

Idaho
76 West 100 North
Blackfoot, ID 83221
208/785-0685

Illinois
8903 Burlington Ave.
Brookfield, IL 60513
708/485-2080
800/284-4442 (Illinois only)

Indiana
4707 E. Washington St. Suite A
Indianapolis, IN 46201
317/356-7722

Iowa
2101 Kimball
Waterloo, IA 50702
319/291-3552
800/475-4442 (Iowa only)

Kansas and
Greater Kansas City
1100 Pennsylvania, Suite 305
Kansas City, MO 64105-1336
816/842-8607
800/783-1356

Kentucky
PO Box 24564
Lexington, KY 40524-4564
502/769-3100

Louisiana
2900 Clearview Park, No. 202
Metairie, LA 70006
504/455-7199

Maine
PO Box 2224
Augusta, ME 04338-2224
207/626-0022

Maryland
916 South Rolling Road
Catonsville, MD 21228
410/747-7758
800/221-6443 (Maryland only)

Massachusetts
Denholm Building
484 Main Street, Suite 325
Worcester, MA 01608
508/795-0244
800/242-0040
(Massachusetts only)

Michigan
8137 W. Grand River, Suite A
Brighton, MI 48116
313/229-5880
800/772-4323 (Michigan only)
FAX: 313/229-8947

Minnesota
12 Colonial Office Park
2700 University Ave., W.
St. Paul, MN 55414
612/644-1121
800/669-6442 (Minnesota only)

Mississippi
PO Box 55912
Jackson, MS 39296-5912
601/981-1021

Missouri
P.O. Box 84
Jefferson City, MO 65102
314/893-2444

Montana
Institute for Health and
Human Services
Eastern Montana College,
Room 235
1500 North Thirtieth St.
Billings, MT 59101-0298
406/657-2077
FAX: 406/761-5110

Nebraska
Route 1, Box 132
Milford, NE 68405
402/761-2781
800/743-4781 (Nebraska only)

Nevada
4074 Autumn Street
Las Vegas, NV 89120
702/454-7666

New Hampshire
2-1/2 Beacon Street
Concord, NH 03301
603/225-8400

New Jersey
1090 King George Post Rd.,
No. 708
Edison, NJ 08837-3722
908/738-1002

New Mexico
2819 Richmond, N.E.
Albuquerque, NM 87107
505/889-8008
800/279-7450
(New Mexico only)

New York
855 Central Ave.
Albany, NY 12206-1506
518/459-7911
800/228-8201 (New York only)

North Carolina
301 South Tryon Street,
Suite 1710
Charlotte, NC 28282
704/332-9834
800/377-1464
(North Carolina only)

North Dakota
P.O. Box 1764
Fargo, ND 58107
701/281-0527
800/279-6344
(North Dakota only)

Ohio
1335 Dublin Rd., Suite 50-A
Columbus, OH 43215-1000
614/481-7100
FAX: 614/481-7130
800/686-5963 (Ohio only)

Oklahoma
PO Box 25011
Oklahoma City, OK 73124
405/556-0147

Oregon
P.O. Box 11295
Eugene, OR 97440-3495
503/689-7310

Pennsylvania
2400 Park Dr.
Harrisburg, PA 17110
717/540-9215
800/245-7443
FAX: 717/657-8265

Rhode Island
Independence Square, 500
Prospect Street
Pawtucket, RI 02860
401/725-2360

South Carolina
P.O. Box 1912
Orangeburg, SC 29116
803/533-1613

South Dakota
Association and Sioux Falls
Area Head Injury
Support Group
221 South Central, Suite 32
Pierre, SD 57501
605/224-0937

Tennessee
PO Box 1090
Hendersonville, TN 37077-1090
615/264-3052

Texas
8911 Capitol of Texas Hwy.
North, Suite 4140, Building 4
Austin, TX 78759
512/794-8688
800/392-0040
FAX: 512/794-0132

Utah
1800 South West Temple,
Suite 208
Salt Lake City, UT 84115
801/484-2240

Vermont
P.O. Box 1837, Station A
Rutland, VT 05701
802/446-3017

Virginia
3212 Cutshaw Ave., Suite 315
Richmond, VA 23230
804/355-5748

Washington, D.C.
2100 May Flower Dr.
Lake Ridge, VA 22192
202/877-1464

Washington State
300 120th Avenue NE
Building 3, Room 131
Bellevue, WA 98005
206/451-0000
800/523-5438 (Washington only)

West Virginia
P.O. Box 574
Institute, WV 25112-0574
304/766-4892
800/356-6443
(West Virginia only)

Wisconsin
735 N. Water Street, Suite 701
Milwaukee, WI 53202
414/271-7463

Wyoming
246 South Center, Suite 206
Casper, WY 82601
307/473-1767
800/244-4636 (Wyoming only)

SELECTED RESOURCES

NATIONAL ORGANIZATIONS AND ASSOCIATIONS

National Head Injury Foundation (NHIF)
1776 Massachusetts Avenue, N.W., Suite 100
Washington, D.C. 20036
202/296-6443
Helpline: 800/444-6443

JMA Foundation, Inc.
National Brain Injury Research Foundation
1612 K Street, N.W., Suite 204
Washington, D.C. 20006
202/331-8445
800/929-0491

European Brain Injury Society (EBIS)
17 Rue de Londres
1050 Brussels, Belgium
322/502.34.88
FAX: 322/514.47.73

**International Association for the Study of Tramatic Brain Injury
(IASTBI)**
PO Box 7019
Columbia, MO 65212-7017
314/882-6786
314/882-3101
FAX: 314/884-4540

Brain Information Service (BIS)
University of CA Brain Information Sciences
Center for Health Sciences
Los Angeles, CA 90024
310/825-3417
310/206-3499

National Institute on Neurological Disorders and Stroke (NINDS)
9000 Rockville Pike, Building 31, Room 8A16
Bethesda, MD 20892
301/496-5751
301/402-2186

Society for Cognitive Rehabilitation
PO Box 33548
Decatur, GA 30033-0548
404/939-6338
404/491-6746

The Perspectives Network
9919 Orangevale Drive
Spring, TX 77379-5103
713/251-7005
713/251-7005

A Comprehensive Model of Research and Rehabilitation for the Traumatically Brain Injured
Medical College of Virginia
MCV-Box 677
Richmond, VA 23298-0677
804/371-2374
TDD: 804/786-0956
FAX: 804/371-2378

A Comprehensive System of Care for Traumatic Brain Injury
Institute for Medical Research
Santa Clara County
950 S. Bascom Avenue, Suite 2011
San Jose, CA 95128
408/295-9896
408/287-9447

A Model System for Minimizing Disability after Head Injury
The Institute for Rehabilitation and Research
1333 Moursund Avenue
Houston, TX 77030
713/799-5000
713/797-5790
713/668-5210

Model Project for Comprehensive Rehabilitation Services to Individuals with Traumatic Brain Injury
Mt. Sinai Medical Center, School of Medicine
One Gustave L. Levy Place
New York, NY 10029-6574
212/241-9657
212/348-5901

South Eastern Michigan Traumatic Brain Injury System
Wayne State University Medical Center
Rehabilitation Institute of Michigan
Detroit, MI 48202
313/745-9769
313/745-1175

RESEARCH AND TRAINING CENTERS

Research and Training Center for Community Integration of Persons With Traumatic Brain Injury
State University of New York at Buffalo
194 Farber Hall, 3435 Main Street
Buffalo, NY 14214
716/829-2300

Research and Training Center on Head Trauma and Stroke
New York University Medical Center
400 East 34th Street
New York, NY 10016
212/263-6161
FAX: 212/263-7190

Rehabilitation Research and Training Center on Severe Traumatic Brain Injury
Medical College of Virginia/Virginia Commonwealth University
MCV Box 434
Richmond, VA 23298-0434
804/786-7209
TDD: 804/786-0956
FAX: 804/371-6340

Research and Training Center in Traumatic Brain Injury
University of Washington
Department of Rehabilitation Medicine
BB-919 Health Sciences Building
Seattle, WA 98195
206/543-6766
FAX: 206/685-3244

Pediatric Research and Training Center
University of Connecticut Health Center
Department of Pediatrics
Division of Child & Family Studies
The Exchange, Suite 164
170 Farmington Avenue
Farmington, CT 06032
203/674-1485

Research and Training Center to Improve Services for Seriously Emotionally Handicapped Children and Their Families
Portland State University
Regional Research Institute for Human Services
P.O. Box 751
Portland, OR 97207-0751
503/464-4040

COMMUNITY LIVING

Research and Training Center for Community Integration of Persons with Traumatic Brain Injury
State University of New York (SUNY) at Buffalo
194 Farber Halla, 3435 Main Street
Buffalo, NY 14214
716/829-2300
TDD: 716/829-3007
FAX: 716/829-2390

Research and Training Center on Residential Services and Community Living
Institute on Community Integration
College of Education
University of Minnesota
214 Pattee Hall, 150 Pillsbury Drive, S.E.
Minneapolis, MN 55455
612/624-6328
TDD: 612/624-7003
FAX: 612/624-9344

Research and Training Center on Community Integration
Resource Support
Syracuse University, Center on Human Policy
724 Comstock Avenue
Syracuse, NY 13244-4230
315/443-3851

INDEPENDENT LIVING

ILRU Research and Training Center in Independent Living
at TIRR
The Institute for Rehabilitation and Research
1333 Moursund Avenue
Houston, TX 77030
713/799-7011

Research and Training Center on Independent Living
University of Kansas, Bureau of Child Research
3111 Haworth Hall
Lawrence, KS 66045
913/864-4095

TRAUMATIC BRAIN INJURY

Research and Training Center on Improving Supported Employ-
ment Outcomes for Individuals with Developmental and Other
Severe Disabilities
Virginia Commonwealth University School of Education
VCU Box 2011
Richmond, VA 23284-2011
804/367-1851
TDD: 804/367-2494
FAX: 804/367-2193

Trauma Center Impact on the Disability Outcomes of Brain and
Sprinal Cord Injury Survivors
National Rehabilitation Hospital
102 Irving Street, N.W.
Washington, D.C. 20010-2949
202/675-2600
FAX: 202/675-2610

OTHER RESOURCES

American Coalition of Citizens with Disabilities
1346 Connecticut Avenue, N.W.
Room 308
Washington, D.C 20036
202/785-4265

Beach Center on Families and Disability
c/o Life Span Institute
3136 Haworth Hall
The University of Kansas
3136 Haworth
Lawrence, KS 66045
913/864-7600
913/864-7605

Center for Children with Chronic Illness and Disability
University of Minnesota
Box 721 - UMHC
Harvard Street at East River Road
Minneapolis, MN 55455
612/626-2398
612/624-3939 Voice and TDD

Coma Recovery Association
377 Jerusalem Avenue
Hempstead, NY 11550
516/486-2847

A Chance to Grow
3820 Emerson Ave., North
Minneapolis, MN 55412
612/521-2266

Family Survival Project
Caregiver Resource Center
425 Bush Street, Suite 500
San Francisco, CA 94108
415/434-3388
800/445-8106 (in CA)

Medical Research and Training Center in Rehabilitation and Childhood Trauma
Tufts-New England Medical Center
Department of Rehabilitation Medicine
750 Washington Street, Box 75K/R
Boston, MA 02111
617/956-5031

National Aphasia Association
PO Box 1887
Murray Hill Station
New York, NY 10156--611

National Spinal Cord Injury Association
600 West Cummings Park, Suite 2000
Woburn, MA 01801
800/962-9629
617/935-2722

Paralyzed Veterans of America
801 18th Street, N.W.
Washington, D.C. 20006
202/USA-1300

The Phoenix Project
Box 84151
Seattle, WA 98124
206/329-1371

**The President's Committee on Employment of People
with Disabilities**
1331 F Street, N.W., Suite 300
Washington, D.C. 20004
202/376-6200

World Institute on Disability
510 Sixteenth Street, Suite 100
Oakland, CA 94612-1502

ABLEDATA Database Program
(Database of Commercial Products for Use in All Aspects of
Independent Living)
8455 Colesville Road, Suite 935
Silver Spring, MD 20910
800/346-2742
FAX: 301/587-1967

SELECTED BOOKS AND PERIODICALS RELATED TO HEAD INJURY, DISABILITY, AND THE FAMILY

BOOKS

Life Beyond the Classroom, Edited by P. H. Wehman, Baltimore. Published by Paul H. Brookes, 1993

National Directory of Lecturers and Resources in Traumatic Brain Injury, Rehabilitation Research & Training Center on Severe Traumatic Brain Injury, MCV Box 434, Richmond, VA 23298-0434.

Applications and Outcomes of Behavior Analysis and Brain Injury Rehabilitation: Basic Principles, by H. Jacobs. Gaithersburg, MD. Published by Aspen Publishers, 1993.

Sexuality and the Person with Traumatic Brain Injury: A Guide for Families, by E. R. Griffith. Philadelphia. Published by F. A. Davis Co., 1993.

Academic Recovery After Head Injury, by D. Russell. Springfield, IL. Published by C. C. Thomas, 1992.

Awareness of Deficit After Brain Injury: Clinical and Theoretical Issues, edited by G. P. Prigatano and D. L. Schacter. New York. Published by Oxford University Press, 1991.

Rehabilitation with Brain Injury Survivors: An Empowerment Approach, by C. C. O'Hara and M. Harrell. Gaithersburg, MD. Published by Aspen Publishers, 1991.

Head Injury: A Family Matter, by J. Williams and T. Kay. Published by Paul H. Brookes, 1991.

Cognitive Rehabilitation for Persons with Traumatic Brain Injury: A Functional Approach, by J.S. Kreutzer and P.H. Wehman. Published by Paul H. Brookes, 1991.

Treating Families of Brain-Injury Survivors, by P.R. Sachs. Published by Springer, 1991.

Work Worth Doing: Advances in Brain Injury Rehabilitation, by B.T. McMahon and L.R. Shaw. Published by PMD Publishers Group, Inc., 1991.

The Psychological and Social Aspects of Disability, by R.P. Marinelli and A.E. Dell Orto. Published by Springer, 1991.

Clinical and Neuropsychological Aspects of Closed Head Injury, by J. Richardson, New York. Published by Taylor & Francis, 1990.

Parenting a Child with Traumatic Brain Injury, by B. K. Hughes, Springfield, IL. Published by C. C. Thomas, 1990.

Traumatic Brain Injury and Neuropsychological Impairment: Sensorimotor, Cognitive, Emotional, and Adaptive Problems of Children and Adults, by R. S. Parker. New York. Published by Springer-Verlan, 1990.

Vocational Rehabilitation for Persons with Traumatic Brain Injury, edited by P. Wehman and J. S. Kreutzer. Rockville, MD. Published by Aspen Publishers, 1990.

Rehabilitation of the Adult and Child with Traumatic Brain Injury (2nd ed.), edited by M. Rosenthal. Philadelphia. Published by Davis, 1990.

Community Integration Following Traumatic Brain Injury, by J.S. Kreutzer and P.H. Wehman. Published by Paul H. Brookes, 1990.

Vocational Rehabilitation for Persons with Traumatic Brain Injury, edited by Paul Wehman, Ph.D. and Jeffrey S. Kreutzer, Ph.D. Published by Aspen, 1990.

Rehabilitation of the Adult and Child with Traumatic Brain Injury. Edited by M. Rosenthal, E.R. Griffith, M.R. Bond & J.D. Miller. Published by F.A. Davis, Philadelphia, 1990.

Assessment of the Behavioral Consequences of Head Trauma. Edited by Lezak, New York. Published by Alan R. Liss, 1989.

Traumatic Brain Injury, by P. Bach-y-Rita. Published by Demos; 1989.

Disability and the Family: A Guide to Decision for Adulthood, by H.R. Turnbull, A.P. Turnbull, G.J. Bronicki, J.A. Summers, and C. Roeder-Gordon, Baltimore. Published by Paul H. Brookes, 1989.

Respite Care: Principles, Programs, and Policies, by S. Cohen and R.D. Warren, Austin. Published by PRO-ED, 1989.

Neuropsychological Treatment of Head Injury, by A. Christensen & D. Ellis, Boston. Published by Martinus Nijhoff, 1988.

Helping the Patient with Brain Injury to Learn: Self-feeding as a Place to Begin. National Institute for Disabilities and Rehabilitation Research, Moss Rehabilitation Hospital, PA, 1988.

Head Injury Rehabilitation: The Role of the Family in TBI Rehabilitation, by M. Guth, Lasseter, S.A. and M. Harward. (Vol. 19 in the HDI Professional Series on Traumatic Brain Injury, edited by W.H. Burke, M. Wesolowski, and W.F. Blackerby, Houston). Published by HDI, 1988.

Family Interventions Throughout Chronic Illness and Disability, by P.W. Power, A.E. Dell Orto and M. Gibbons. Published by Springer, 1988.

Community Re-entry, by J.W.P. Traphagan. Published by the National Head Injury Foundation, Washington D.C., 1988.

The Head-injured College Student, by C.B. Holmes. Published by Charles C. Thomas, 1988.

Chronic Illness and Disability. Edited by Catherine Chilmen, Elan Nunnaly and Fred Cox, Newbury Park, CA. Published by Sage, 1988.

Unending Work and Care: Managing Chronic Illness At Home, by J. Corbin and A. Strauss, San Francisco. Published by Jossey-Bass, 1988.

Rehabilitation of the Severely Brain Injured Adult: A Practical Approach. Edited by I. Fussey and G.M. Giles. Published by Brooks, London, 1988.

Adolescent Community Integration, by J. Fryer. In: National Invitation Conference on Traumatic Brain Injury Research: Vol. 2. Chesepaeake Community Head Injury Center, MD, 1987.

From the Ashes: A Head Injury Self-Advocacy Guide, by C. Miller and K. Campbell, Seattle, WA. Published by The Phoenix Project, 1987

Rehabilitation Psychology Desk Reference, by Bruce Caplan. Published by Aspen, 1987.

A Positive Approach to Head Injury, by B. Slater. Published by Slack, 1987.

Community Re-entry for Head-injured Adults, by M. Ylvisaker and E.M. Gobble. Boston: College-Hill, 1987.

Brain Injury Rehabilitation: A Neurobehavioral Approach, by R.L. Wood, London. Published by Croom Helm, 1987.

Positive Approach to Head Injury: Guidelines for Professionals and Families, by B. Slater, New Jersey. Published by Slack, 1987.

From the Ashes: A Head Injury Self-Advocacy Guide, by C. Miller and K. Campbell. Published by Phoenix Project, Seattle, WA, 1987.

Head Trauma: Educational Reintegration, by C. Rosen and J. Gerring, San Diego. Published by College-Hill, 1986.

Neuropsychological Rehabilitation After Brain Injury, by G.R. Prigatano, Baltimore. Published by Johns Hopkins University Press, 1986.

Family as Therapeutic Agent: Long-Term Rehabilitation for Traumatic Head Injury Patients. Mary E. Switzer Fellowship Report, by H.E. Jacobs. Published by the National Institute of Handicapped Research, 1984.

Closed Head Injury: Psychological, Social and Family Consequences. Edited by N. Brooks. Published by Oxford University Press, Oxford, 1984.

Rehabilitation of the Head Injured Adult, by M. Rosenthal, E.
    Griffith, M. Bond, and J. Miller, Philadelphia. Published F.A.
    Davis, 1983.

The Humpty Dumpty Syndrome, by J. Warrington Moffatt, J.
    Available from the National Head Injury Foundation. 1981.

PERIODICALS

Brain and Cognition
Academic Press, Inc.
1250 6th Avenue
San Diego, CA 92101-4312
619/699-6742
FAX: 619/699-6859

Brain Injury
Taylor & Francis, Ltd.
1900 Frost Road, Suite 101
Bristol, PA 19007-1598
215/785-5800
FAX: 215/785-5515

The Journal of Cognitive Rehabilitation
6555 Carrollton Avenue
Indianapolis, IN 46220
317/257-9672

The Journal of Head Injury
1612 K Street, N.W., Suite 204
Washington, D.C. 20006
800/929-0491

The Journal of Head Trauma Rehabilitaion
Aspen Publishers, Inc.
7201 McKinney Circle
PO Box 990
Frederick, MD 21701-9727
801/698-7100

Mouth: The Voice of Disability Rights
61 Brighton Street
Rochester, NY 14607
FAX: 716/442-2916

NHIF Newsletter
National Head Injury Foundation
1776 Massachusetts Avenue, N.W., Suite 100
Washington, D.C. 20036

D

Selected Films And Videos On Head Injury

Available from:

The Transitional Learning Community at Galveston
Brain Injury Rehabilitation
P.O. Box 1228
1528 Post Office
Galveston, TX 77553
409/762-6661
1-800-TLC-GROW
FAX: 409/762-9961

BROKEN RHYMES
Commentary on brain injury featuring four survivors on their
journey through rehabilitation; 57 minutes.

JOURNEY FROM FLANDERS
Sequel to Broken Rhymes following up on the four survivors of
brain injury from the original film, five years later; 38 minutes.

MENDING OF THE MINDS
Commentary on head injury, rehabilitation and the social responsibility involved; 20 minutes

STORMS IN THE MIND
Overview of the Transitional Learning Community Program, 20
minutes.

Available from:

> PMD Publishers Group, Inc.
> PO Box 4116
> Winter Park, FL 32793
> 407/657-3737
> 800/438-5911
> FAX: 407/657-4499

ASSESSING BRAIN FUNCTION. 20 minutes

COUNSELING TECHNIQUES FOR BRAIN-INJURED CLIENTS WITH LANGUAGE DIFFICULTIES. 8 minutes

COUNSELING TECHNIQUES FOR GIVING NEGATIVE FEEDBACK: SANDWICH TECHNIQUE. 8 minutes

COUNSELING TECHNIQUES FOR WORKING WITH CLIENTS WHO DENY DISABILITY. 10 minutes

COUNSELING TECHNIQUES FOR WORKING WITH THE RIGID AND PERSEVERATIVE CLIENT. 11 minutes

Available from:

> National Head Injury Foundation
> 1776 Massachusetts Avenue, N.W., Suite 100
> Washington, DC 20036
> 202/296-6443

COMA. A 15 minute, five part series exploring the issues and myths surrounding coma. It is an excellent introduction to the complexities of coma and its effect on families. Includes scenes from a very poignant and emotional support group meeting.

A FATE BETTER THAN DEATH. An 18 minute tape featuring four young adults with head injuries. Focuses on support groups and the comments of families as they cope with the magnitude of problems caused by head injuries.

SURVIVING COMA: THE JOURNEY BACK. A 57 minute documentary that originally aired on Public Broadcast Stations, this is an inspiring look at head injury and its consequences. Includes an in-depth look at euthanasia through one case study.

SURVIVING COMA: THE JOURNEY BACK. A 19 minute version of "Surviving Coma: The Journey Back" with less emphasis on euthanasia and more emphasis on traumatic brain injury and prevention.

THE UNSEEN INJURY: MINOR HEAD TRAUMA. A two video educational package suitable for survivors, family members, and professionals (57 minutes). Five copies of the professional brochure and 20 copies of the family brochure accompany the two tapes.

THE UNSEEN INJURY: MINOR HEAD TRAUMA. A 20 minute segment of the 2 part series, "The Unseen Injury," designed specifically for viewing by family members. Single copies of the family and professional brochure accompany the tape.

Available from:

> Rehabilitation Research and Training Center on Severe
> Traumatic Brain Injury
> Medical College of Virginia
> Virginia Commonwealth University
> Box 434
> Richmond, VA 23298-0434
> 804/786-7290

THE EFFECTS OF HEAD INJURY ON THE FAMILY.

ETHICAL ISSUES FOR FAMILIES OF TBI PATIENTS.

FAMILY PERSPECTIVES ON HEAD INJURY.

THE IMPACT OF BRAIN INJURY ON RELATIONSHIPS: THREE PERSONAL STORIES

MANAGEMENT OF THE AGGRESSIVE PATIENT.

REBUILDING RELATIONSHIPS AFTER TRAUMATIC BRAIN INJURY.

SEXUALITY ISSUES FOLLOWING TRAUMATIC BRAIN INJURY: A PHYSIATRIC PERSPECTIVE.

WHY CAN'T PATIENTS THINK STRAIGHT?

Available from:

> Rehabilitation Research & Training Center
> Community Integration of Persons with TBI
> State University of New York at Buffalo
> 194 Farber Hall
> 3435 Main Street
> Buffalo, NY 14214
> 716/829-2300

LIVING WITH THE EFFECTS OF TRAUMATIC BRAIN INJURY: THREE HISPANIC FAMILIES (In Spanish with English subtitles).

PROBLEMS AND COPING STRATEGIES OF MOTHERS, SIBLINGS AND YOUNG ADULT MALES WITH TRAUMATIC BRAIN INJURY.

E

An Educational Program For Families Of Persons With Head Injury– A Practical Application Of Head Injury And The Family: A Life and Living Perspective

Introduction

This program is designed for family members who are living with the daily reality of head injury. The program itself utilizes selected material which has been presented in varied chapters of this book. The sessions of this program are developed to take place after the person's in-hospital treatment. Stressors on the family may interfere with information processing during the acute phase of hospitalization, and effective family education may take place when the person is undergoing rehabilitation. The different sessions are designed to be presented in flexible time formats. For example, the program could be presented in the evenings, on weekends, or at other times more appropriate to the needs of the family members.

Assumptions

In planning the content of the workshop, different assumptions are used as guidelines for program development:

1. As described in Chapter 3, the needs of the family needs change during treatment and rehabilitation. During the acute care phase family members may show shock, denial, and even panic, and when the person returns to consciousness, there is both a sense of relief and almost a massive denial of the implications of head

injury for future life functioning. Eventually, as the family realizes that certain behavioral and cognitive functions may not return to pre-injury levels, the denial slowly breaks down to be replaced by anger, grief, and depression. All of these emotions give rise to distinct needs, such as the needs for support, information, and the acquisition of management skills. But after a number of months, following head injury onset, these needs may be highlighted, combined with other needs. These needs, which are identified below, form the basis for much of the program content:

- family support
- special social opportunities
- special therapies (e.g., cognitive rehabilitation)
- learning how to deal with management concerns
- financial assistance
- job training/work programs

2. When planning a family education program, family members should be provided with opportunities for new learning, including the beginning acquisition of special skills.

3. The educational program should also provide opportunities for family networking and support. Frequently, the real benefit from family participation is acquiring new friends or the growing awareness that others are experiencing similar difficulties.

4. During each session, family members should have the opportunity in a group atmosphere to process the information communicated by the presenters with other family members. In this atmosphere, guidelines should be observed, such as confidentiality, the encouragement of questions, an option to pass (Don't have to comment), members should be supportive, and a focus on "I" statements.

5. Information related to head injury should be provided in an integrated format, and this communication should assist in the prevention of further problems during the recovery period that may inhibit eventual life or vocational adjustment.

6. Family members who have successfully coped with head injury should be included as presenters.

WORKSHOP OBJECTIVES

At the end of the workshop, the family members should:

1. Gain an understanding about the complexity of a head injury.
2. Begin to understand their own emotions.
3. Learn effective management techniques.
4. Become aware of resources.
5. Begin to understand what recovery from head injury involves.
6. Learn to deal with caregiving responsibilities.
7. Begin to receive and give support.

FIRST SESSION

Goal: To help participants identify their own family problems resulting from living with a person with head injury. Participants should have read highlights of Chapter 1.
Materials: Copies of the chapter highlights, blackboard, pencils, paper.

EDUCATIONAL PLAN

1. After providing copies of the highlights of Chapter 1, presenter should ask participants to read it, looking specifically for implications for their own family life.

2. Presenter should discuss briefly the main points of Chapter 1 and emphasize what could be the many family problems resulting from living with a person with head injury.

3. Individuals/family members will break into small groups. (There will be a recorder for each group.) The group will:
   a. read Set #5 and discuss it
   b. discuss personal implications of Chapter 1
   c. highlight any family problems and suggest possible solutions

4. Break/social when refreshments are served.

5. Each group gives its report, identifying the problems most people feel they have encountered, and some of the suggestions in resolving the problems. The presenter may then wish to provide a brief summary.

SECOND SESSION

Goal: To help participants understand the implications of head injury on the injured member's life functioning. Participants should have read a handout that identifies the highlights of Chapter 2.
Materials: Copies of the highlights and Set #6, blackboard, pencils, paper.

EDUCATIONAL PLAN

1. After providing copies of Chapter 2 highlights, presenter should ask participants to read it. Presenter should also identify varied symptomology of the person during the recovery period, and what are some management problems.

2. Individuals/family members will break into small groups. (There will be a recorder for each group.) The group will:
   a. Read Set #6 and discuss it
   b. Discuss management problems and suggest possible solutions

3. Break/social when refreshments are served

4. Each group gives its report, identifying the management problems and possible suggestions for resolution. The presenter may then wish to provide a brief summary.

THIRD SESSION

Goal: To help participants understand the family implications of head injury, and to become aware of effective coping skills to deal with family problems. Participants should have read a handout that identifies the highlights of Chapter 3.
Materials: Copies of the chapter highlights, Set #11, pencils, and paper.

EDUCATIONAL PLAN

1. Review chapter. Presenter should discuss such coping strategies as stress monitoring, reframing, how to identify family reinforcements and how to get in touch with family strengths.
2. Break into groups.
   a. read Set #11 and discuss
   b. discuss coping strategies

3. Break/social.

4. Large group give report; presenter summarize.

FOURTH SESSION

Goal: To help family members deal with many of their losses and grief resulting from head injury. Participants should read handout that identifies the highlights of Chapter 8.
Materials: Copies of Chapter 8 highlights, Set #13, blackboard, pencils, and paper.

EDUCATIONAL PLAN

1. Presenter will review chapter highlights with participants. Participants will underline points of personal interest in the chapter. Presenter may wish to discuss personal losses related to head injury and coping approaches.

2. Break into groups.
   a. read Set #13 and discuss
   b. discuss coping strategies

3. Break/social

4. Give reports in large group; presenter summarize material.

FIFTH SESSION

Goal: To help family members utilize community resources and continue networking with other families. Participants should read a separate handout identifying highlights of Chapters 9 and 10.
Materials: Copies of handout, Set #14, blackboard, pencils, and paper.

EDUCATIONAL PLAN

1. Presenter should review highlights of Chapters 9 and 10, and then identify and discuss community resources and networking possibilities within one's own geographic area.

2. A panel of family caregivers will discuss their utilization of community resources and invite feedback and questions from the workshop participants.
3. Break/social

4. Presenter will summarize all the material discussed and invite participants to continue their interaction with each other.

To be noted:

- include the importance of utilizing assertive skills when discussing community resources.
- community resources should also include vocational rehabilitation.
- speakers from community organizations could be invited to participate.

INDEX

INDEX

A

Abuse of alcohol, and head injury, 140, 173-185
    violence with, 180
Acceptance
    as emotional reaction, to head injury, 26, 60, 195
    therapeutic approach to, by family, 106-108
Adaptive patterns, of family members, 64-65
Adjustment
    of family members
        acceptance of individual with brain injury, 60
        age of individual with brain injury, at time of injury, 63-64
        chronic stress, 61
        communication skills, 60
        damage to family relationships, appraisal of, 77
        empathy, exercise in, 68-69
        family strengths, 58-61
        interpersonal functioning, inadequacy of, 61-62
        lack of information, 62
        lingering grief, 63
        listening ability, 58
        maladaptive patterns, 64
        negative sick role expectations, 62-63
        negotiation ability, 59
        positive reinforcement, 59-60
        present orientation, 59
        problems in, 57-69
        responsibility-taking ability, 58
        self-caretaking ability, 59
        sexual concerns, 63

shared perception of reality, 58
social isolation, 63
transgenerational coping strategies, presence of, 60-61
styles of, pre-injury, 89
Age, of individual with brain injury
and adjustment, of family members, 63-64
empathy, exercise in, 52
impact on coping with, 22-23
Aggressive behavior, of brain-injured individual, 9, 160
Alcohol abuse, 173-185
group counseling, 140
violence with, 180
Aloneness, of trauma center experience, 4
Ambiguity, ability to cope with, 23
Ambivalence, inability to express, as obstacle in grieving
process, 125
Assessment, of family members, 73-83
adjustment, to head injury, damage to family relationships, 77
communication patterns, 75
demographic information, 74-75
division of labor, 75
family relationship, health of, 77
guidelines for, 74-77
head injury characteristics, 76
and health issues, 76
impact of head injury on family, 76-77
and outside socialization of family, 76
Assumptions
about family support, held by health care system, 4-5
theoretical, in family intervention, 88-96
At-Home Rehab Program, of Michael W. Bales, Sr., 8-12

B

Background, cultural, of family, 40
Bales, Michael W., Sr., At-Home Rehab Program, 8-12
Belief system, testing of, 6
Bereavement, in family of brain-injured individual, 121-135
Blame, within family, of individual with brain injury, 40-41
Body image, if individual with brain injury, 21
Burnout, of caregiver, and respite care, 160

C

Cash settlement, payment of, for head injury, emotional issues
          regarding, 195-196
Causes, of brain injury, 20
Center, trauma, experience, aloneness of, 4
Centrality, term usage, 124
Children's group model, group counseling, 144
Chronic stress, and adjustment, of family members, 61
Common perception of reality, and adjustment,
          of family members, 58
 Communication
      and adjustment, of family members, 60
      patterns, and family assessment, 75
Competence, sense of, and family intervention, 90
Concept of "normal life", after head injury, 11-12
Coping
      resources, of family, 39
      style, of individual with brain injury, 25
Counseling
      and family intervention, 92-93
      group, 139-152
            children's group model, 144
            didactic group model, 144
            family group model, 144
            female group model, 144
            financial pressure issues, 141
            job loss issues, 140
            leadership of group, 141-143
            male group model, 144
            marital group model, 144
            marital relationship issues, 140
            medical staff group, 144
            multidimensional model, 143-145
            neglect of family unit members, issues regarding, 140
            peer group model, 144
            quality of life group model, 144
            relatives, removal of support issues, 141
            sibling acting-out issues, 140
            sibling group model, 144
            significant other model, 144
            spousal group model, 144
            substance abuse issues, 140
            theme group model, 144
            vocational rehabilitation group model, 144

Crisis intervention, for family of brain-injured individual, 106-109
    beginning phase, 106-107
    middle phase, 107-108
    termination phase, 109
Crying, inability, as obstacle in grieving process, 125
Cultural background, of family, 40
Cure, traumatic brain injury, issues regarding, 13

D

Demographic information, for family assessment, 74-75
Denial
    as emotional reaction, to head injury, 24
    and family of individual with brain injury, 42-43
    as obstacle in grieving process, 125
Depression, as emotional reaction, to head injury, 24-25
Design, of health care system, inadequacy of, 3-4
Diagnosis, of alcoholism, with head injury, 177
Didactic group model, group counseling, 144
Division of labor, and family assessment, 75
Drug abuse, group counseling, 140

E

Education, and family intervention, 93-95
Emotional reaction, to head injury, 23-26
    acceptance, 26
    coping style, 25
    denial, 24
    depression, 24-25
    grieving, 24
    guilt, 25
    homecoming experience, 27-32

F

Family
    belief system, testing of, 6
    crisis, helping approach, 106-109
        beginning phase, 106-107
        middle phase, 107-108
        termination phase, 109
    grief of, 121-135
    group model, of group counseling, 144
    head-injured individual, importance of each, 14

interaction, 38
    reaction of, to individual with brain injury, 22
    sense of loss, experienced by, 121-135
Family assessment, 73-83
    communication patterns, 75
    and damage resulting from adjustment to head injury, 77
    demographic information, 74-75
    division of labor, 75
    guidelines for, 74-77
    and head injury characteristics, 76
    and health issues, 76
    and health of family relationship, 77
    and impact of head injury on family, 76-77
    and outside socialization of family, 76
Family intervention, 87-100
    caregiver skill, teaching techniques, 89
    counseling and, 92-93
    and education, 93-95
    illness, in addition to head injury, 99-100
    joint venture approach, 88
    normalization of family relationships, 90-91
    past adjustment styles, 89
    quality of life, and rehabilitation focus, 89
    sense of competence, imparting of, 90
    strengths, increasing awareness of, 91
    stress points, 88-89
    support and, 95-96
    theoretical assumptions, 88-96
Female
    group model, group counseling, 144
    as respite care provider, issues regarding, 159
Financial resources. *See also* Payment
    effect on emotional burdens, 7
    loss of, group counseling, 140-141
Frame of reference, realism of, effect on coping, 6-7
Friends, removal of support, as group counseling issue, 141

G

Gender issues, in respite care, 159
Goal flexibility, and bereavement intervention, 124
Grief
    ambivalence, inability to express, as obstacle in process, 125
    centrality, term usage, 124
    crying, inability, as obstacle in, 125
    denial, as obstacle in, 125
    as emotional reaction, to head injury, 24
    of family of brain-injured individual, 43, 121-135

goal flexibility, of family of brain-injured individual, 124
inability to express unresolved feelings regarding past losses,
    as obstacle in grieving process, 125
intense reaction of, understanding, 123-124
intervention approach, in family's grieving process, 125-128
lingering, and adjustment, of family members, 63
obstacles to progress in, 124-125
peripheral, term usage, 124
preventable, term usage, 124
resentment, inability to express, as obstacle in process, 125
self-knowledge, of health-care professional, and bereavement
    intervention, 122
stages of, and bereavement intervention, 122
unpreventable, term usage, 124
Group counseling, 139-152
children's group model, 144
didactic group model, 144
family group model, 144
female group model, 144
financial pressure issues, 141
job loss issues, 140
male group model, 144
marital group model, 144
marital relationship issues, 140
medical staff group, 144
multidimensional model, 143-145
neglect of family unit members, issues regarding, 140
peer group model, 144
quality of life group model, 144
relatives, removal of support issues, 141
sibling acting-out issues, 140
sibling group model, 144
significant other model, 144
spousal group model, 144
substance abuse issues, 140
theme group model, 144
vocational rehabilitation group model, 144
Guidelines, for family assessment, 74-77
Guilt
as emotional reaction, to head injury, 25
within family, of individual with brain injury, 40-41

H

Head injury
adjustment of family, 57-70
alcohol, effect of, 173-189
assessment of family, 73-83

characteristics, and family assessment, 76
grief process, 121-135
group counseling, 139-152
impact on family, 37-53
impact on person, 19-34
intervention, 87-135
life care plan, 200-201
loss, 121-135
monetary compensation settlement issues, 200-201
myths regarding, 194-197
overview, 3-15
respite care, 155-170
resuscitation by trauma team, ramifications of, 199-200
withholding medical care, at accident scene, 199-200
Health issues, and family assessment, 76
Health of family relationship, and family assessment, 77
History, of familial interaction, 4-5
Homecoming experience, of individual with brain injury, 27-32

I

Illness, in addition to head injury, and family intervention, 99-100
Impact, of head injury
    on family, 37-53
        blame, 40-41
        coping resources, 39
        cultural background, 40
        denial, 42-43
        determinants of, 37-41
        grief, 43
        guilt, 40-41
        interaction of family, 38
        life cycle of family, 39
        meaning of injury to family, 38
        patterns of family reaction, 41-45
        pre-injury relationship to injured person, 39-40
        previous crises, reaction to, 38
        re-orientation process, 43-44
        realization process, 43
        shock, 42
        stressors, nature of, 41
        support system availability, 40
    on injured person, 19-34
        body image, 21
        emotional reaction, 23-26
            acceptance, 26
            coping style, 25
            denial, 24

depression, 24-25
grieving, 24
guilt, 25
familial reaction, 22
homecoming, 27-32
life stages, 22-23
location of injury/lesion, 23
personality makeup of individual, 20-21
philosophy of life, 22
previous satisfaction, 21
religion, 22
societal reaction, 22
therapeutic intervention, 22
uncertainty, ability to live with, 23
Importance of individual with brain injury, balanced with
        family's importance, 14
Inadequacy of health care system design, 3-4
Inadequacy of interpersonal functioning, and adjustment, of
        family members, 61-62
Information, lack of, and adjustment, of family members, 62
Intense grief reaction, understanding of, 123-124
Intervention
    family, 87-100
        caregiver skill, teaching techniques, 89
        counseling and, 92-93
        education and, 93-95
        and illness, in addition to head injury, 99-100
        joint venture approach, 88
        normalization of family relationships, 90-91
        past adjustment styles, 89
        quality of life, and rehabilitation focus, 89
        sense of competence, imparting of, 90
        strengths, increasing awareness of, 91
        stress points, 88-89
        support and, 95-96
        theoretical assumptions, 88-96
        therapeutic, for individual with brain injury, 22

J

Job loss issues, group counseling, 140
Joint venture approach, to family intervention, 88

L

Lack of information, and adjustment, of family members, 62
Leadership, of group, in group counseling, 141-143
Life cycle
    of family unit, and head injury timing, 39
    of individual with brain injury, 22-23
Lingering grief, and adjustment, of family members, 63
Listening ability, and adjustment, of family members, 58
Location, of brain injury/lesion, impact of, 23
Loss, sense of, in family of brain-injured individual, 121-135

M

Maladaptation, of family, to chronic illness, of individual with brain
    injury, 64
Male group model, group counseling, 144
Marital group model, group counseling, 144
Marital relationship issues, group counseling, 140
Meaning of head injury, to family, 38
Medical intervention, helpfulness of, issues regarding, 196-197
Medical staff group, group counseling, 144
Missouri Head Injury Association, 10
Monetary resources. *See also* Payment
    effect on emotional burdens, 7
    loss of, group counseling, 140
Multidimensional group counseling model, 143-145
Myths, regarding head injury, 194-197

N

National Head Injury Foundation, establishment of, 5
Negative sick role expectations, and adjustment,
    of family members, 62-63
Neglect of family unit members, group counseling, 140
Negotiation, and adjustment, of family members, 59
"Normal life", concept of, after head injury, 11-12
Normalization of family relationships, and family
    intervention, 90-91

O

Obstacles, to progress in grieving, 124-125
Outside socialization of family, and family assessment, 76

P

Past adjustment styles, family intervention, 89
Past losses, inability to express unresolved feelings regarding,
    as obstacle in grieving process, 125
Patterns of family reaction, to chronic illness, 41-45
Payment
    for care of individual with brain injury, 14
    of cash settlement, for head injury, emotional issues
    regarding, 195-196
Peer group model, of group counseling, 144
Peripheral, term usage, 124
Personality, of individual with brain injury, before injury, 20-21
Philosophy of life, of individual with brain injury, 22
Positive reinforcement, and adjustment, of family members, 59-60
Pre-injury activities, satisfaction with, of individual with
                brain injury, 21
Pre-injury personality, of individual with brain injury, 20-21
Present orientation, and adjustment, of family members, 59
Preventability of head injury, myth regarding, 194-195
Preventable, term usage, 124
Previous crisis, family reaction to, 38

Q

Quality of life
    group model, group counseling, 144
    and rehabilitation focus, in family intervention, 89

R

Re-orientation process, and family of individual with brain
                injury, 43-44
Reaction, of family, to individual with brain injury, 22
Realization process, and family of individual with brain injury, 43
Relationship, to individual with brain injury, pre-injury, 39-40
Relatives, removal of support, as group counseling issue, 141
Religion, of individual with brain injury, 22

Resentment, inability to express, as obstacle in grieving
        process, 125
Respite care, 155-170
    and aggressive behavior of brain-injured individual, 160
    and caregiver burnout, 160
    and change in role, with head injury, 161
    defined, 156-157
    family need overview, 157-159
    gender issues and role, 159
    recognition of need for, 155-156
    role flexibility and, 159
    sharing of caregiving burden, 168
Responsibility-taking ability, and adjustment, of family
        members, 58
Role
    change in, with head injury, 161
    flexibility, and respite care, 159
    of individual with brain injury, within family, 39

S

Satisfaction, with activities pre-injury, of individual with
        brain injury, 21
Self-caretaking ability, and adjustment, of family members, 59
Self-knowledge, of health-care professional, and bereavement
        intervention, 122
Sexual concerns, and adjustment, of family members, 63
Shared perception of reality, and adjustment, of family
        members, 58
Sharing, of caregiving burden, respite care and, 168
Shock, of family of individual with brain injury, 42
Sibling acting-out issues, group counseling, 140
Sibling group model, group counseling, 144
Sick role expectations, negative, and adjustment, of
        family members, 62-63
Significant other model, group counseling, 144
Social isolation, and adjustment, of family members, 63
Society, reaction of, to individual with brain injury, 22
Spivack, Marilyn Price, National Head Injury Foundation,
        establishment of, 5
Spousal group model, group counseling, 144
Stage
    of family life cycle, and head injury timing, 39
    of grief process, and bereavement intervention, 122
Status, of individual with brain injury, within family, 39
Strengths, increasing awareness of, and family intervention, 91
Stress
    chronic, and adjustment, of family members, 61

nature of, to family, 41
     points, and family intervention, 88-89
Substance abuse issues, group counseling, 140
Support, in family intervention, 40, 95-96

T

Tantrums, of injured individual, 9, 160
Testing, of belief system, 6
Theme group model, group counseling, 144
Theoretical assumptions, in family intervention, 88-96
Therapeutic intervention, for individual with brain injury, 22
Time frame, severe head trauma, 13
Transgenerational coping strategies, presence of, and adjustment,
     of family members, 60-61
Trauma. *See* Head injury

U

Uncertainty, ability to cope with, 23
Unpreventable, term usage, 124

V

Violence, and alcohol abuse, 180
Vocational rehabilitation group model, group counseling, 144
Vulnerability, of family, to unforeseen events, 6-7

W

Withholding of care, to head-injured accident victim, 200
Work performance, deterioration of, as group counseling issue, 140